THE STORY OF BRITAIN'S
BLACK NURSES

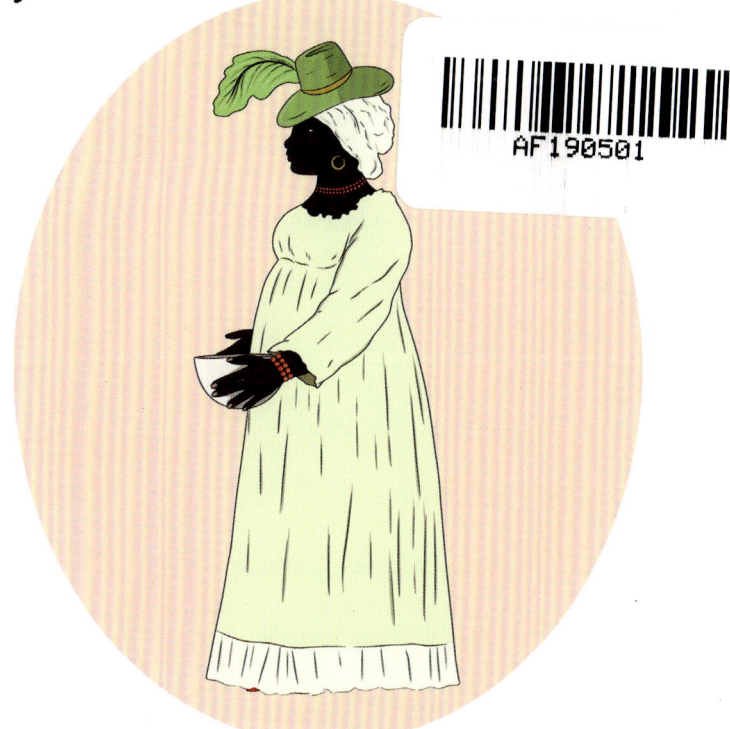

K.N. CHIMBIRI

ILLUSTRATED BY
SIMONE DOUGLAS AND JAEL UMERAH MAKELEMI

SCHOLASTIC

CONTENTS

When you come across words in **bold**, turn to page 66 to find their definitions in the glossary.

INTRODUCTION

In Britain today, there are hundreds of thousands of nurses. Nurses are trained to take care of people at different stages of their lives, from newborn babies to the elderly. They often work in hospitals alongside doctors and other healthcare workers. Some work in private homes, schools or care homes. Others work only with children while some work with adults.

The story of Britain's Black nurses also includes countries outside Britain. This may seem surprising today, but Britain once had an enormous **empire**, and ruled a vast network of countries that included **colonies** all around the world. Some of those colonies were in Africa. Others were in the North Atlantic Ocean such as Bermuda and many islands in, or near, the Caribbean Sea. The empire also included countries on the American mainland such as Canada, British Guiana (Guyana) and British Honduras (Belize).

This story of Britain's Black nurses includes many incredible nurses from these places.

TODAY, MOST NURSES ARE

WOMEN, BUT THROUGHOUT

HISTORY, THERE HAVE **ALWAYS**

BEEN **MEN** IN NURSING.

"I LIKE NURSING BECAUSE IT IS **NOT SELFISH**. THAT IS I DO NOT HELP MY FAMILY ALONE BUT **EVERYONE IN NEED OF HELP** – WHETHER WHITE, BLACK OR ANY OTHER RACE."

MIRIAM MULONGE
AS RECORDED IN
THE ZAMBIA NURSE
JOURNAL, 1965

CHAPTER ONE

ANCIENT AND MEDIEVAL AFRICA

Throughout history, people have cared for other people. Today, in our highly organized society we have doctors, nurses, **pharmacists** and other healthcare specialists. In the past, it wasn't always like this. Sometimes doctors prepared medicines themselves. Sometimes nurses decided how to treat their patients and they made recipes for medicines.

Our ancient ancestors studied nature and tested remedies. They noticed what medicines worked and could develop their body of knowledge. In some societies the information was written down. In others it was passed down by word of mouth.

The ancient Egyptians created a long-lasting, organized civilization. It was based on religion and they believed in making offerings to their gods to help solve health problems. However, they also used natural remedies, such as plants, minerals and animal products, to heal.

They made **mummies** using linen bandages, oils, herbs and **natron** to preserve the skin and organs. They also knew how to use bandages to help people with injuries.

Some of the oldest writings about healthcare come from ancient Egypt. They knew about at least 700 different plant, mineral and animal materials to use as medicines.

Like the ancient Egyptians, people in other parts of Africa also knew about different substances to use as medicine. In West Africa, they used a wide range of plants, relying on the knowledge they had learned over thousands of years. In 1722, a European in the Gold Coast (today's Ghana) noted that the people used herbs '… in Pharmacy, as well as in **Surgery**' and that they 'succeed in many good Cures in both.'

People have always had to fight diseases. **Smallpox** was a highly **infectious disease** – for thousands of years it claimed millions of lives throughout the world. A number of West African peoples invented a treatment to prevent smallpox before the Europeans. In the 1720s, many lives were saved during the smallpox epidemic in the British colony of Boston, New England, because an enslaved African called Onesimus had taught the treatment to his enslaver.

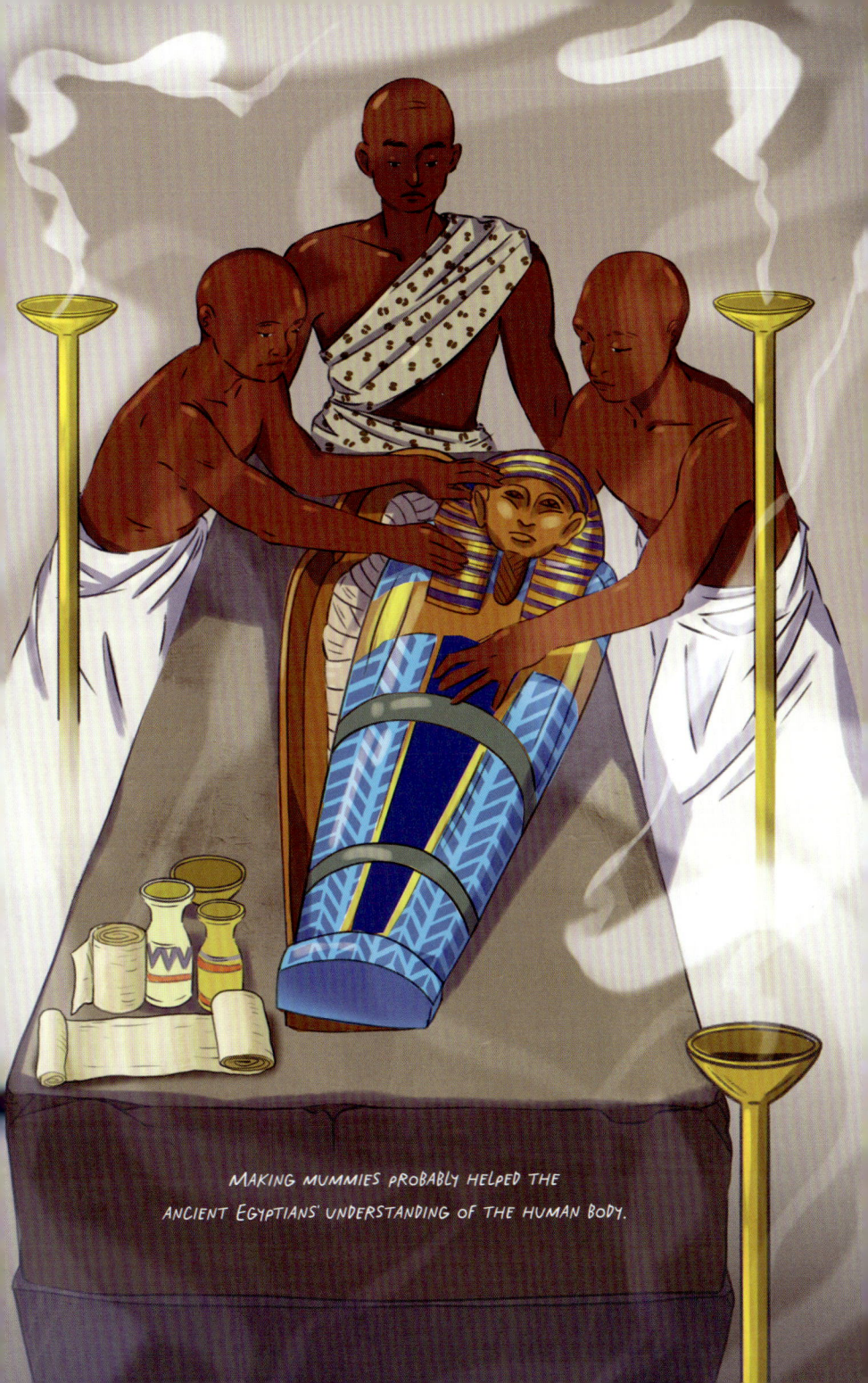

MAKING MUMMIES PROBABLY HELPED THE ANCIENT EGYPTIANS' UNDERSTANDING OF THE HUMAN BODY.

"A GOOD NURSE HAS TO BE **KIND,**

COMPASSIONATE, UNDERSTANDING,

A **GOOD LISTENER,** AND ABLE TO

EMPATHIZE WITH A PATIENT."

BARBARA (DAVIS) WADE
(1936–2006)

FIRST BLACK PERMANENT PUBLIC WARD NURSE AT
KING EDWARD VII MEMORIAL HOSPITAL, BERMUDA

CHAPTER TWO

EUROPE COMES TO AFRICA

In 1492, a European called **Christopher Columbus** sailed to the **Americas** on behalf of Spain. Columbus planned to sail from Europe to Asia. Instead, he landed in the Bahamas! This sparked the beginning of countries in western Europe racing each other to build huge global empires.

The Spanish and Portuguese were the first European nations to claim colonies in the Americas. Later on, the Netherlands, Britain and France became the main colonizers. Over time, Britain, like several other European nations, enslaved millions of people from Africa. It was partly how Britain built up its empire.

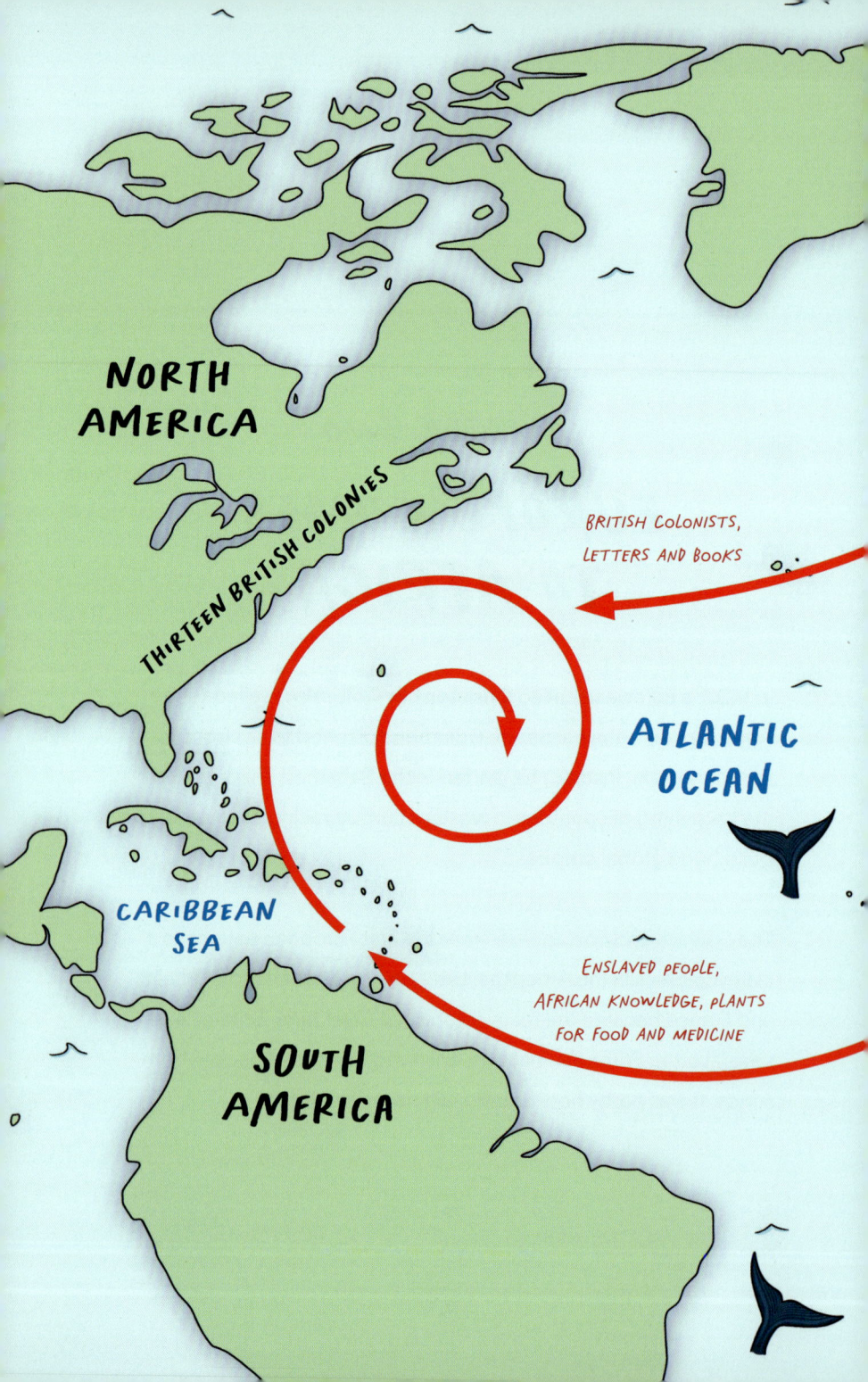

NORTH
AMERICA

THIRTEEN BRITISH COLONIES

BRITISH COLONISTS,
LETTERS AND BOOKS

ATLANTIC
OCEAN

CARIBBEAN
SEA

ENSLAVED PEOPLE,
AFRICAN KNOWLEDGE, PLANTS
FOR FOOD AND MEDICINE

SOUTH
AMERICA

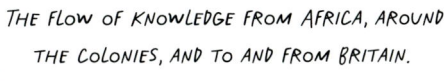

GREAT BRITAIN

EUROPE

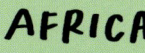

AFRICA

Most of the enslaved people were taken from West and West Central Africa. Millions of people died or were murdered whilst being taken from their homes to the Americas.

People were kidnapped and marched to the coast of West Africa. They were imprisoned before being taken by ship across the Atlantic Ocean in crowded, unhygienic conditions.

Not all of the Africans enslaved by the British were sent to its colonies in the Americas. A small number of enslaved men and women were kept in forts along the West African coast. They were forced to work using their skills, talents and knowledge of traditional African medicine to take care of their enslavers.

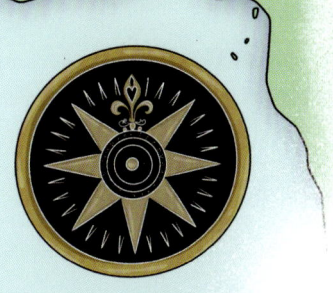

"I HAVE COME TO APPRECIATE NURSING MORE AND MORE AS I'VE GROWN OLDER ... THE ABSOLUTE DEVOTED CARE AND ATTENTION THAT I RECEIVED FROM NURSES AT ALL LEVELS HAS MADE ME ETERNALLY GRATEFUL AND APPRECIATE WHAT IT IS REALLY TO BE CARED BY NURSES."

BERENICE 'BEN' DOLLY
(1917–2002)
NURSE LEADER, TRINIDAD

CHAPTER THREE

CARING DURING ENSLAVEMENT

When the enslaved men, women and children arrived in the British colonies, they were sold to new enslavers who forced them to work without pay, usually on **plantations**. Some were forced to work on sugar plantations. Others were forced to grow and harvest other crops such as coffee and tobacco. Some were made to work in salt ponds or in forests, cutting down trees.

Some enslavers owned big plantations and lived lavish, frivolous lifestyles with plenty of feasts and parties. The enslaved lived much less comfortably. They had to endure poor working and living conditions. Many of them were under-fed, poorly dressed and overworked. They were often harshly punished by their enslavers, particularly if they tried to run away.

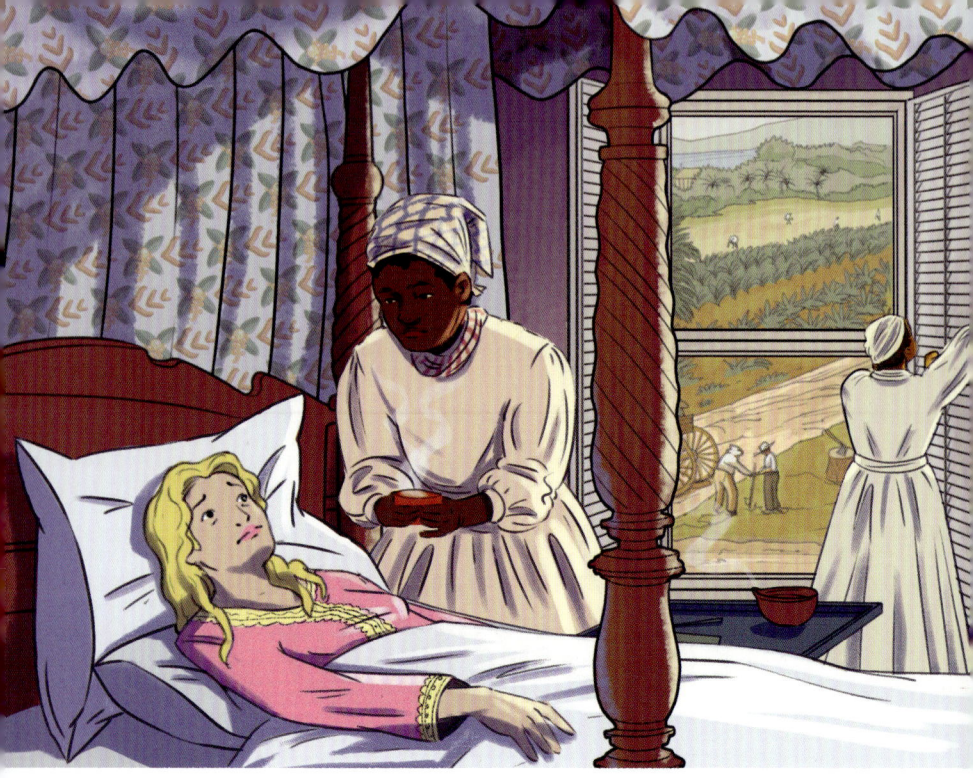

Disease and ill-health could affect everyone in the colonies but the enslaved workers suffered the most.

The enslavers made some of the workers cook, clean and nurse them. They had to take care of their enslavers and their families when they were sick. Both enslaved men and women worked as '**sick-nurses**'. Sometimes they used African methods to treat their enslavers.

Following an African style of medicine, enslaved nurses used herbs and plants to treat illnesses. They made 'bush teas' and used natural treatments. Sometimes these methods worked and they were less harmful than the European treatments at the time.

Medical knowledge was poor compared to today. People didn't understand the causes of diseases and how they spread. It was commonly believed that disease and **epidemics** were a punishment from God for wickedness. Only quite recently have people started to understand the causes of disease.

In 1711, a European in Jamaica recorded that the plant called Majoe Bitters was named after an enslaved woman called Majoe. He wrote that Majoe used the plant to cure 'the most stubborn diseases', which even the 'skilful' European doctors had given up on as their medicine didn't work.

Although the enslaved Africans came from tropical (hot) countries, many of the plants in the Americas were different from the plants in Africa. We will probably never know how the enslaved people figured out how to correctly use some of these plants.

" WITHIN THE NURSING PROFESSION THERE CAN BE NO TIME FOR PREJUDICE, FOR DISEASE KNOWS NO MAN-MADE BARRIERS, NEITHER DOES IT RECOGNIZE SUCH FACTORS AS RACIAL, RELIGIOUS, OR ETHNIC ORIGINS."

MABEL KEATON STAUPERS (1890–1998)

BARBADOS-BORN US CIVIL RIGHTS ACTIVIST AND NURSE, USA

CHAPTER FOUR

CREATING A 'NEW' WORLD

The societies created by the British in their colonies in the Americas were built on the enslavement of Africans and people descended from Africans. Although not all white people were wealthy, and some were mistreated by more powerful white people, white people were not enslaved.

People from Africa were regularly brought to the colonies as enslaved workers. Over time, mixed-race people were born in the colonies. Some mixed-race people were given their freedom by their white fathers, and together with any Black people who had also been freed, were called the free 'people of colour'.

The free 'people of colour' formed a group in between the white people and the enslaved workers. A few free 'people of colour' became wealthy and some even owned enslaved people.

Although they were legally free, the mixed-race and Black people in this middle group did not enjoy the same rights as white people.

The enslaved workers were at the bottom of society. This group was the largest and was made up of Black people and the many mixed-race people who had not been freed by their white fathers. Enslaved people were considered property that could be bought and sold. Children born to enslaved mothers were also considered property.

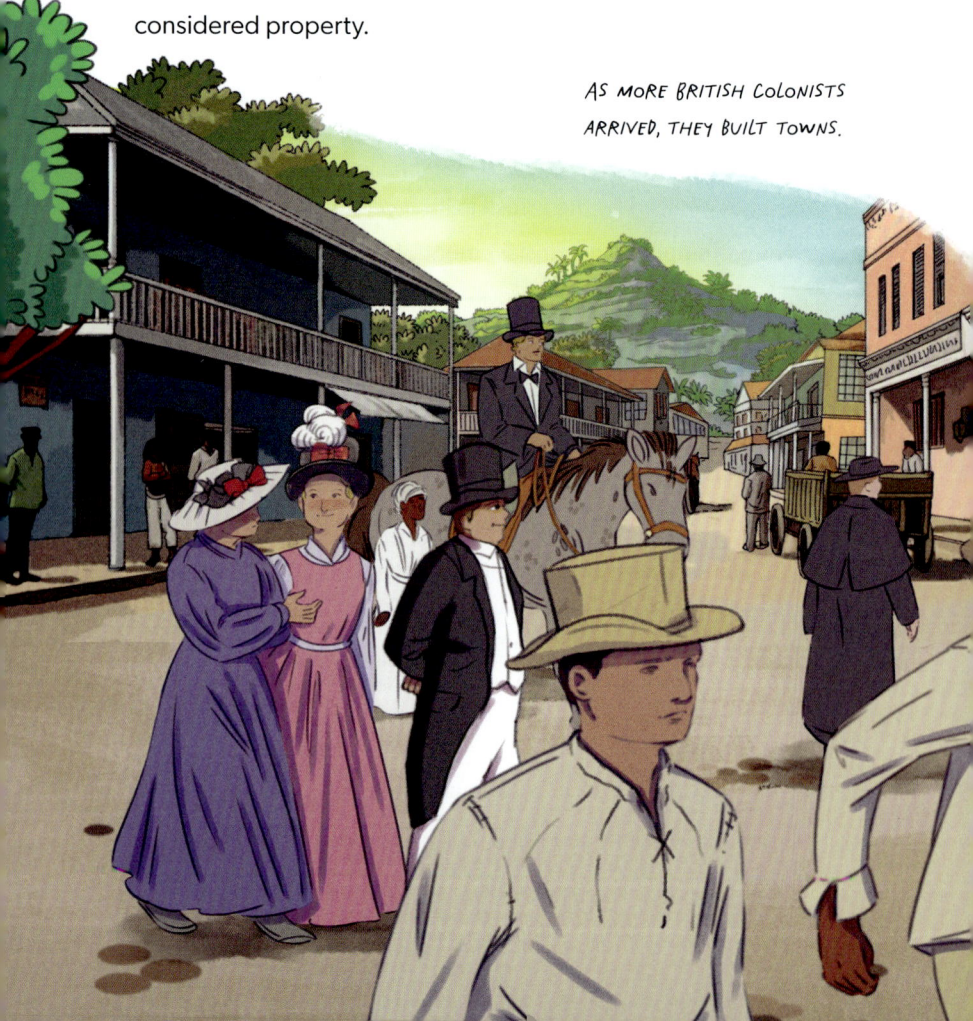

AS MORE BRITISH COLONISTS ARRIVED, THEY BUILT TOWNS.

CHAPTER FIVE

ENSLAVED NURSES

There were doctors in the British colonies, but the enslaved people could not depend on them. Today, we know that anyone from any background can become a doctor or a nurse, but during this period (the 17th and 18th centuries), the doctors in Britain and its colonies were expected to be white men. British society did not view men and women as equals and women of any background were not allowed to become doctors.

Doctors rode around on horseback, or by horse and buggy, to visit the enslavers, their families and the enslaved workers. Their services weren't free and some enslavers did not want to pay for doctors to treat their enslaved workers. Some doctors were enslavers themselves.

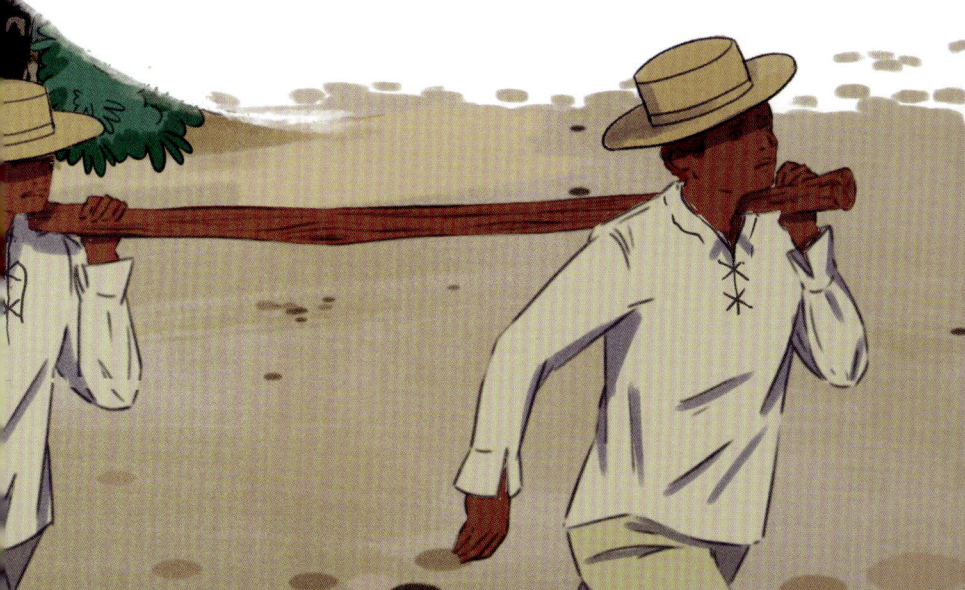

British people, like many other Europeans at the time, did not yet understand the link between hygiene and disease. Almost 2,000 years earlier, when Britain was a part of the Roman Empire, bathing was a part of the culture. Romans, rich or poor, tried to bathe regularly (although they didn't understand that contaminated water could carry disease, or how important it was to keep wounds clean to avoid infection). After the fall of Rome, over time, bathing fell out of fashion in Britain. **Sanitation** in cities like London was also poor.

A doctor, who was also an enslaver, wrote that the enslaved workers should be allowed to bathe in fresh water and then oil their skins in palm oil as most Africans did on the coast back in Africa. He also advised that all plantations should have a sick-house and that the nurse should not be, as they often were, an elderly woman. Enslavers often forced their oldest enslaved woman, who could not do any other work, to be the nurse.

A growing **abolition movement** in Britain alerted the British public to the horror and brutality of enslavement in their colonies. The movement put some pressure on planters to provide hospitals for their enslaved workers but not everyone followed the rules. Some 'sick-houses' were just squalid rooms and some even doubled up as jails. One enslaver on the island colony of Antigua wanted his plantation manager to imprison the enslaved nurse in the hospital at night so she wouldn't try to escape.

ALTHOUGH SOME PLANTATIONS WERE BIG, MOST PLANTATION
HOSPITALS WERE ONLY TWO SMALL UNCLEAN ROOMS.

Nursing in Britain and the empire was not a recognized profession like it is today. On a small plantation the enslaved nurse might have many things to do, including cooking, delivering babies and looking after sick patients and giving them medicine. On some plantations the sick-nurse was a house servant as well.

Nurses were also expected to guard their patients in case they tried to escape. Enslaved people tried to win their freedom in many ways: for example, by pretending to be ill in the hope of trying to escape from an unlocked or unguarded sick-house.

Despite these harsh conditions, some enslaved nurses cared about their patients. One European writer commented that enslaved nurses always mixed arrowroot dishes with great care to make nourishing food for their patients.

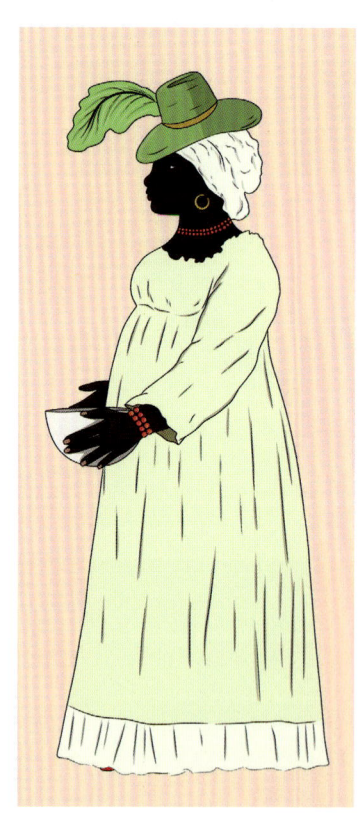

NURSE FLORA WAS AN ENSLAVED WOMAN IN JAMAICA WHO HELPED LADY MARIA NUGENT DURING THE BIRTH OF HER FIRST CHILD. LADY NUGENT WAS WARY OF THE CHARMS AND HERBS, WHICH NURSE FLORA SUGGESTED WOULD HELP WITH CHILDBIRTH.

CHAPTER SIX

THE STORY OF COUBA CORNWALLIS

In 1780 the North American colonies, supported by France, Spain and the Netherlands, were fighting a war against Britain for independence. A young English captain, later an admiral, Horatio Nelson took part in a disastrous **expedition** from Jamaica against the Spanish settlements in Nicaragua. On his way back, Nelson became very ill with the dreaded 'yellow jack' fever. He was taken straight to the **lodging-house** of a Black woman named Couba Cornwallis who was famous for saving the lives of many British naval officers. Using her medical skills and 'herbal brews', Couba nursed the young captain back to health.

Nelson went on to become a British hero. Couba later also nursed Prince 'Sailor Billy' William, Queen Victoria's uncle, when he was a sailor stationed in Jamaica. William later became king (William IV).

Although most people of African descent were enslaved at the time, Couba Cornwallis was not an enslaved woman. She belonged to a group of Black nurses who did not work for the enslavers in their homes or in the plantation sick-houses. This group of free Black and mixed-race women were called 'doctresses'. Doctresses used the Caribbean methods of treatment that had developed among the enslaved people on the plantations. These methods combined the knowledge brought from Africa with the practices they saw of the white doctors. A hundred years later, in Victorian times, one of these women – Mary Seacole – would become the most famous Black woman throughout the British Empire.

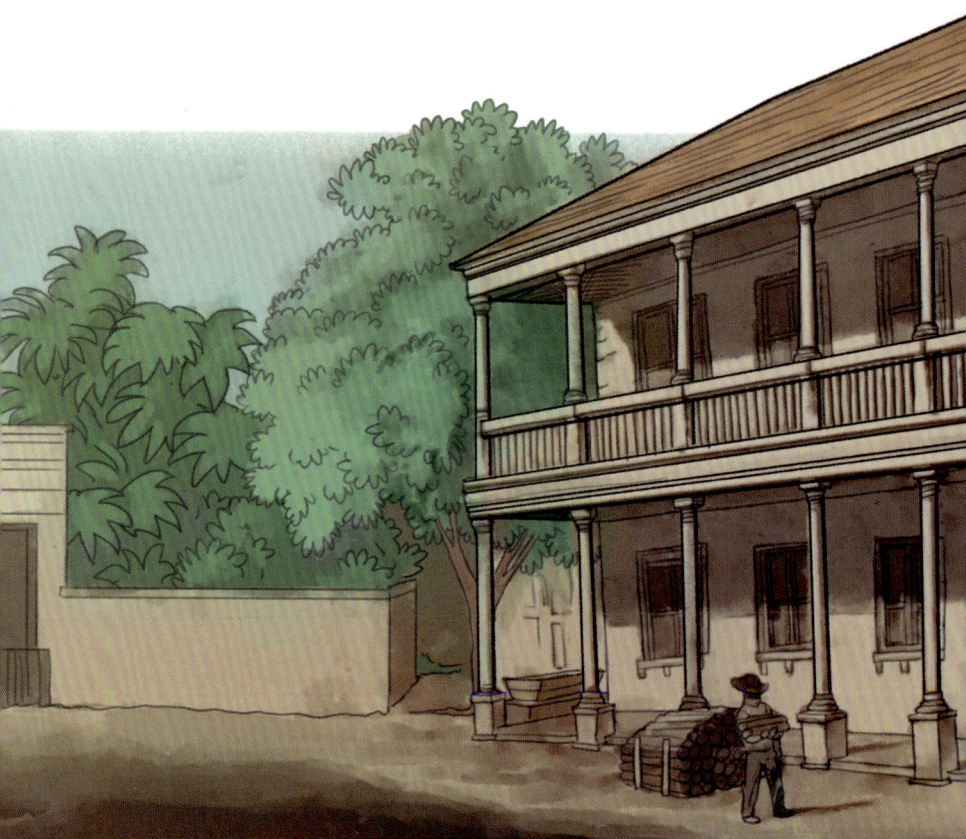

IN THE TOWNS, SOME FREE MIXED-RACE AND BLACK WOMEN COULD OFFER NURSING SERVICES IN LODGING-HOUSES.

"BLACK NURSES WHO FORGED AHEAD IN THE EARLY 1900s **EXEMPLIFIED COURAGE**, **COMMITMENT**, **DEDICATION**, **ASSERTIVENESS**, **ACCOUNTABILITY**, AND AN UNWAVERING BELIEF IN THE **INTEGRITY OF HUMANKIND**. TODAY, BECAUSE OF THESE PIONEERS, BLACK NURSES ARE PRACTISING WITH DIGNITY IN ALL AREAS OF NURSING."

MARY ELIZABETH CARNEGIE (1916–2008)
US NURSE EDUCATOR, AUTHOR AND ACTIVIST

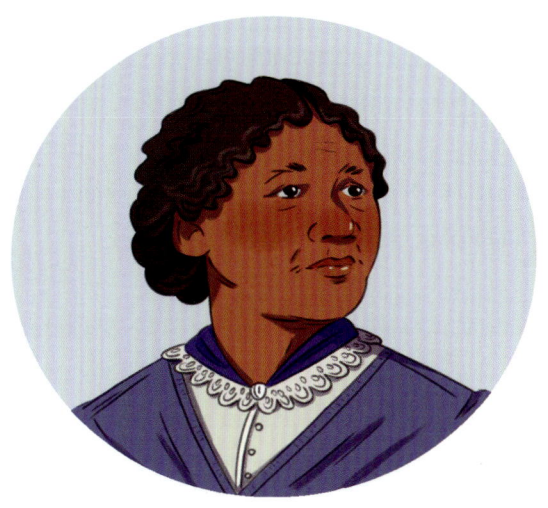

CHAPTER SEVEN

THE STORY OF MARY SEACOLE

Mary Jane Grant was born in 1805 in Jamaica. Mary was born free at a time when most people of colour in the island colony were still enslaved (see chapter 4). Her father was a Scottish army officer and her mother was a mixed-race doctress and lodging-house owner.

Mary belonged to the free 'people of colour' group. Although they were not enslaved, in Jamaica at this time free mixed-race and free Black people were not allowed to vote, do certain jobs or own large amounts of land.

As a child, Mary was taught about herbal treatments, 'doctoring' and nursing by her mother. Mary's mother, like Couba Cornwallis many years before, had a good reputation for her 'doctoring' and nursing skills. By the time she was twelve, Mary was helping her mother tend to patients.

In 1850, while Mary was in Kingston, there was an outbreak of **cholera** and she gained experience treating cholera patients. Mary decided to join her brother who had moved to Panama. Shortly after she arrived, cholera broke out there too. Mary saved her first patient and from then on, rich and poor came to her for treatment. She made sure the sick room was clean, **ventilated** and that patients were kept apart as much as possible. Mary used her natural treatments like 'mustard plasters' and herbal teas. She also learnt how to take care of wounds.

Mary decided to return to Jamaica. In 1853, when there was an outbreak of **yellow fever**, Mary treated patients in her lodging-house. Mary gained a reputation for successfully treating dangerous diseases. She then went back to Panama for a short while.

It wasn't long before Mary started reading about the outbreak of a war in Crimea. British nurses were needed to treat the wounded. Mary had hands-on experience treating cholera, yellow fever and wounds, and thought she could certainly help.

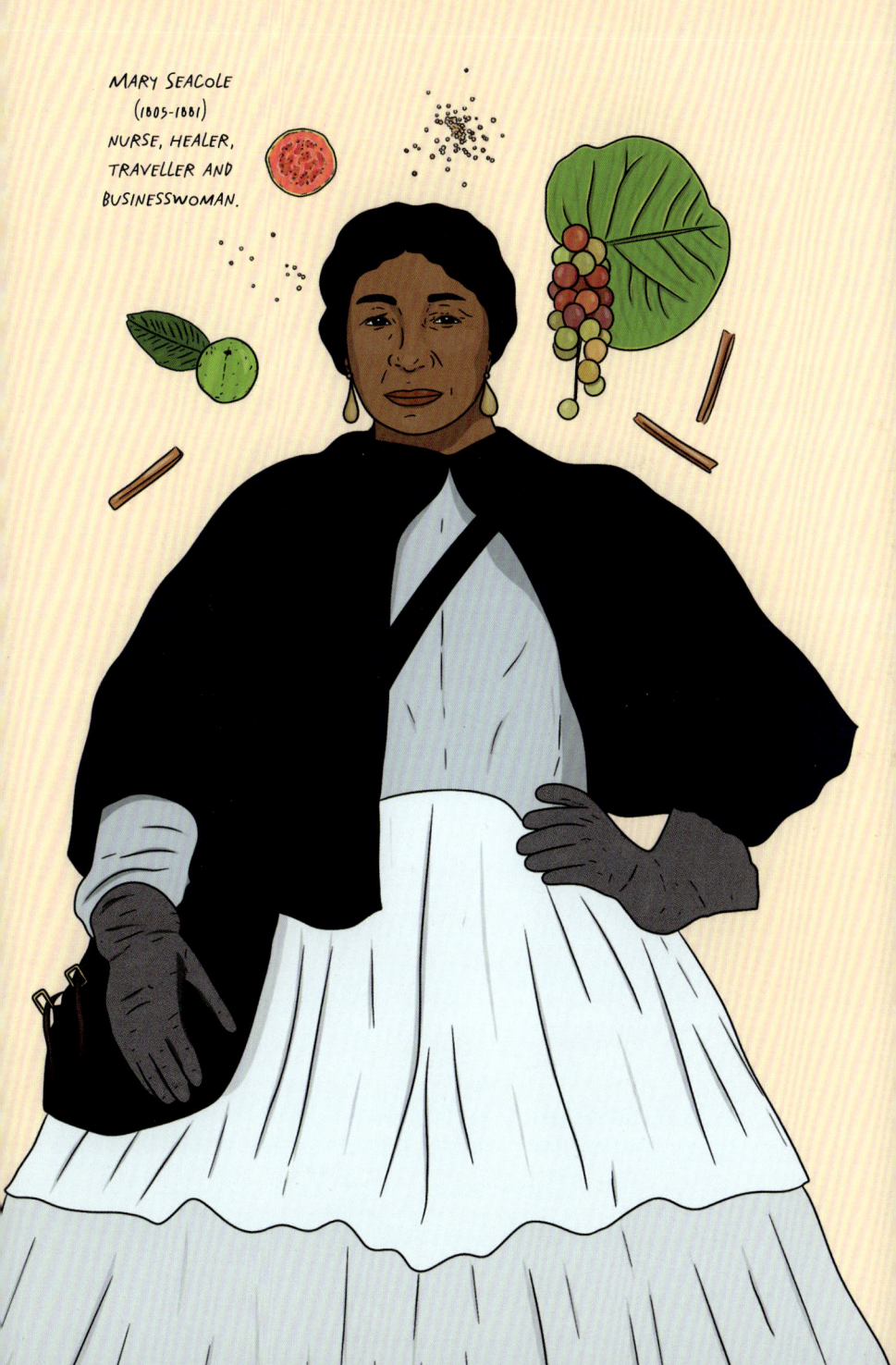

MARY SEACOLE
(1805-1881)
NURSE, HEALER,
TRAVELLER AND
BUSINESSWOMAN.

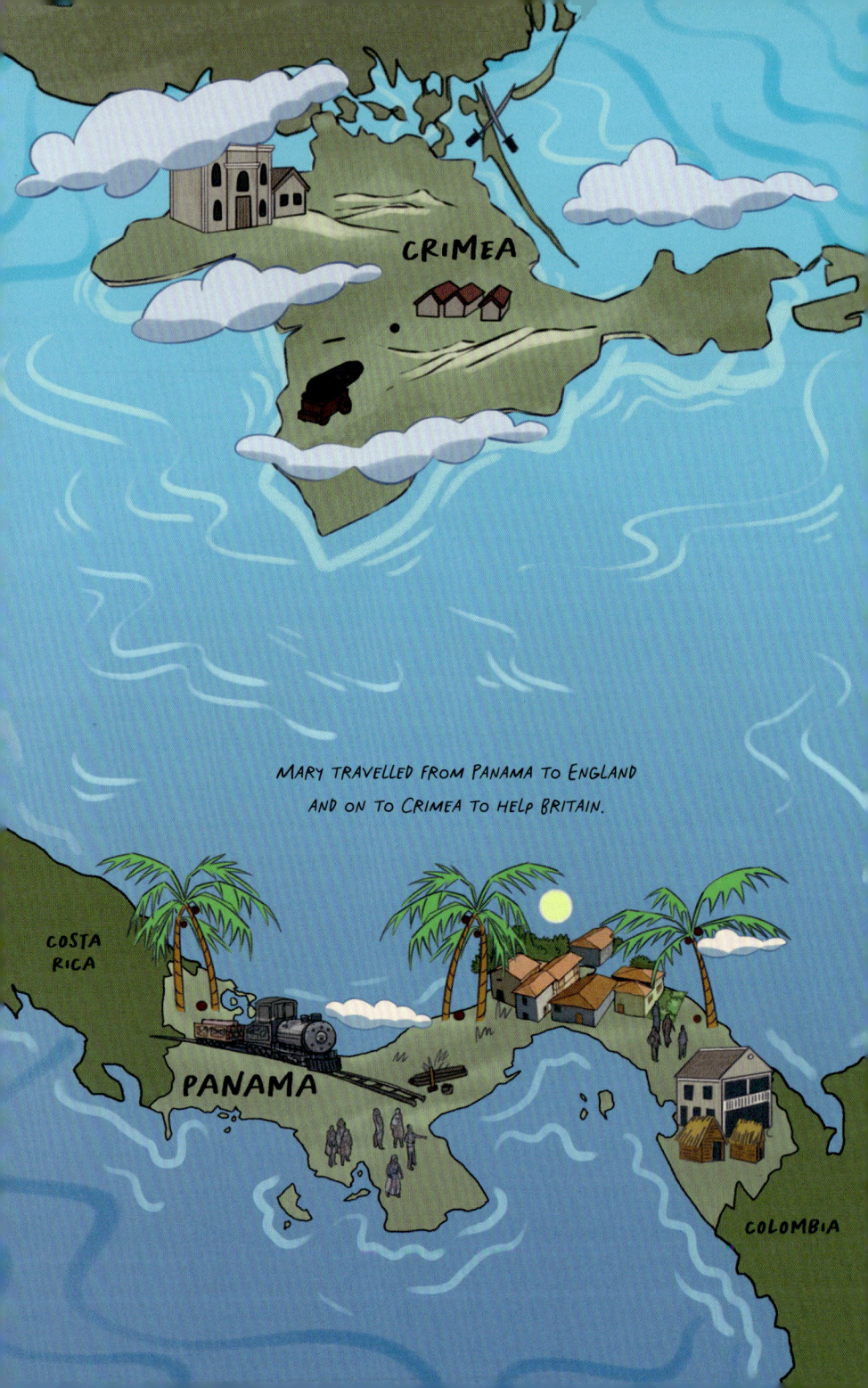

MARY TRAVELLED FROM PANAMA TO ENGLAND
AND ON TO CRIMEA TO HELP BRITAIN.

CHAPTER EIGHT

MARY GOES TO CRIMEA

Turkey and Russia were at war. Russia had invaded Moldavia and Wallachia (in today's Romania), which was part of the Ottoman (Turkish) Empire. Britain, France and later Sardinia entered the war on the side of the Ottomans.

In 1854, Britain and France sent troops to the Crimean Peninsula, which was a part of the Russian Empire. The troops planned to lay **siege** to the Russian naval base at Sebastopol. Although they won battles on the way; on the River Alma, at Balaclava and Inkerman, a mistake by the British **cavalry** at Balaclava caused the deaths of hundreds of men and horses.

The British Army did not have enough food, medicine or suitable clothing for their troops. There was also a lack of doctors, medical supplies and nurses. Thousands of British soldiers were dying from **frostbite**, **malnutrition** and diseases like cholera.

35

More men were dying from disease than from battle injuries. Newspapers, such as the *Illustrated London News* and *The Times*, made the British public aware of the soldiers' suffering. The public demanded action and forced the government to send out women nurses like the French had done.

Mary travelled to London to volunteer as a nurse at the British army hospital but she was turned away. She thought it might have been because she wasn't white. We now know that two other women with African ancestry, Elizabeth Purcell and Miss Belgrave, also volunteered as nurses, but they were turned away because they were not white.

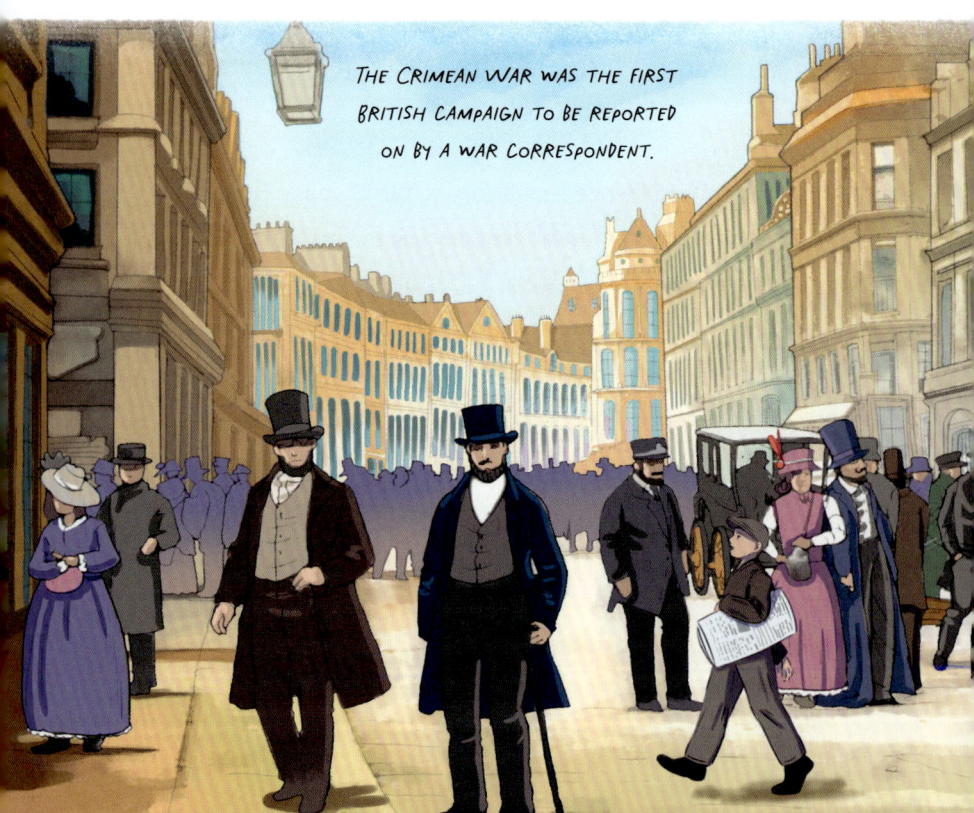

THE CRIMEAN WAR WAS THE FIRST BRITISH CAMPAIGN TO BE REPORTED ON BY A WAR CORRESPONDENT.

Mary was determined to go to Crimea so she made her own way. Once there, she set up her 'British Hotel' near the front lines. It was a general store, canteen and unofficial surgery. Mary served good food for the ordinary soldiers in the canteen, while the officers (who belonged to the upper classes) had an area to relax in the main building. Although Mary sold her goods for 'heavy prices', she nursed for free and was paid for her medicines.

Mary's fame spread because of her successful treatments and 'many acts of comforting kindness'. Newspapers printed stories about Mary and her bravery taking food, drink and medicine to soldiers on the battlefield.

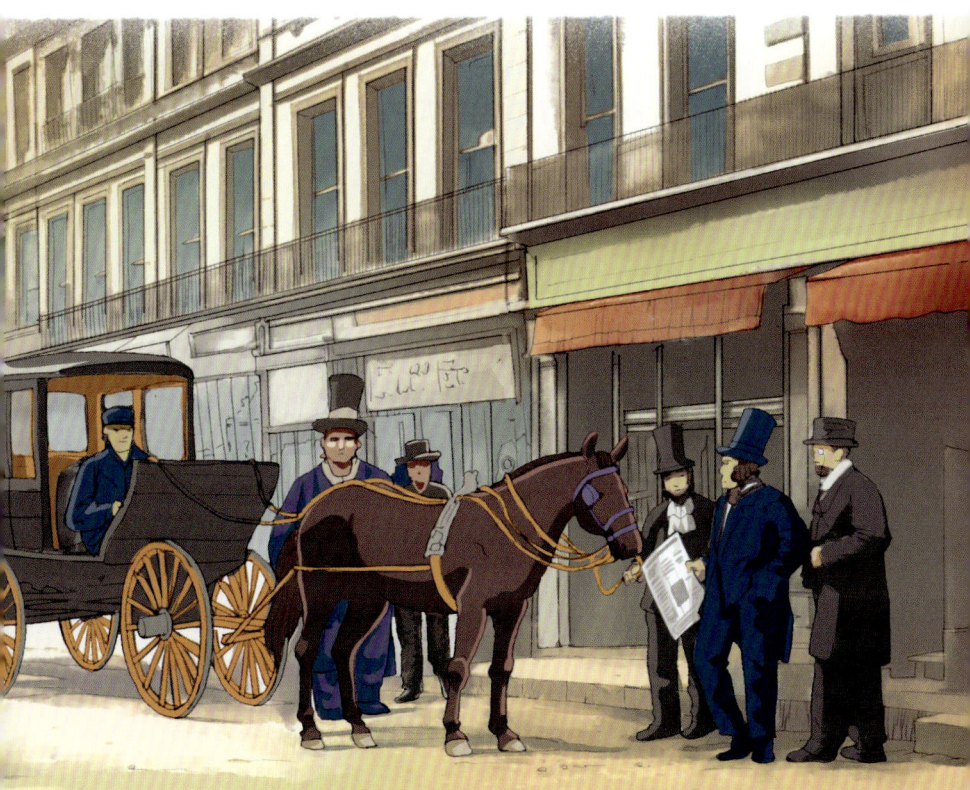

When the war ended suddenly, Mary was left with goods she could no longer sell. Some of the officers hadn't paid their bills. On her return to England, the newspapers reported that she was **bankrupt**. Mary had helped so many of the soldiers in Crimea – now it was their chance to help her.

One veteran recalled:

"BUT FOR THIS LITTLE WOMAN I WOULD NOT BE HERE TODAY. HER NURSING SAVED MY LIFE IN THE CRIMEA."

A fundraising appeal was set up for her as well as a Seacole Festival at the Royal Surrey Gardens. Despite the huge public response, Mary didn't receive much of the money raised for her.

Mary wrote a book about her travels and adventures. It was called *Wonderful Adventures of Mrs Seacole in Many Lands*. Mary's book was published in 1857 and became an instant bestseller.

William Howard Russell, *The Times* reporter, wrote the **preface**:

'… I have witnessed her devotion and her courage. I have already borne testimony to her services to all who needed them … I trust that England will not forget one who nursed her sick, who sought out her wounded to aid and succour them …'

Mary died in London in 1881. She was remembered in Jamaica but forgotten in Britain until 1973 when Jamaican nurses began retelling her story, bringing Mary's tale back to life. And, in 1984, her book was republished for the first time in 127 years.

ON 30 JUNE 2016, A MEMORIAL STATUE OF MARY SEACOLE WAS UNVEILED IN THE GARDENS OF ST THOMAS'S HOSPITAL, LONDON.

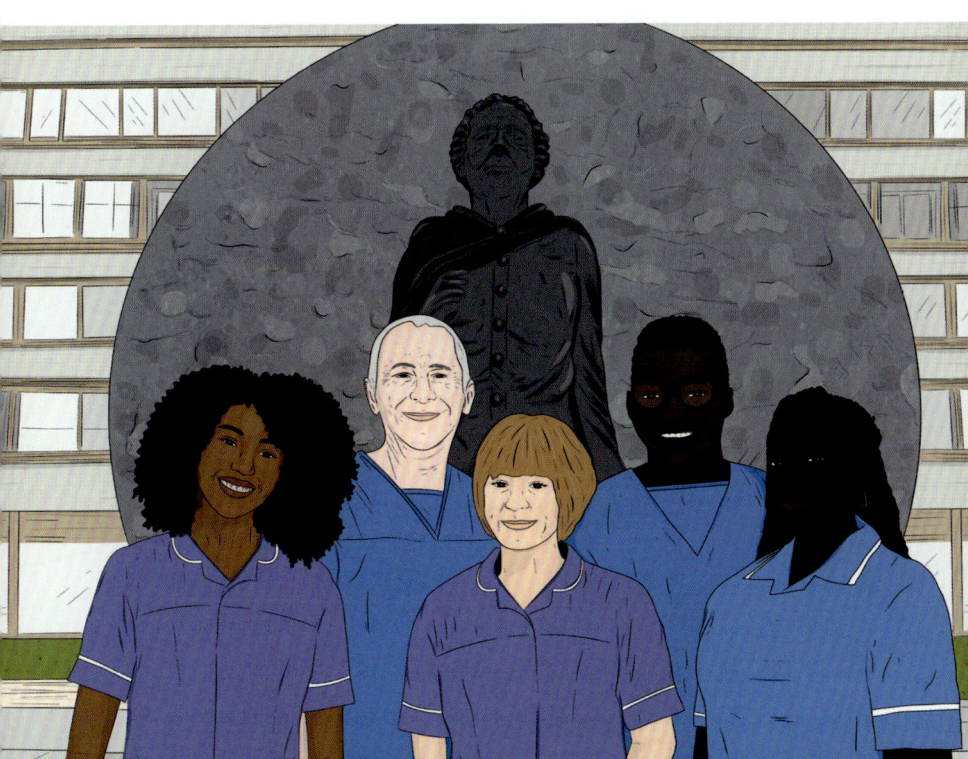

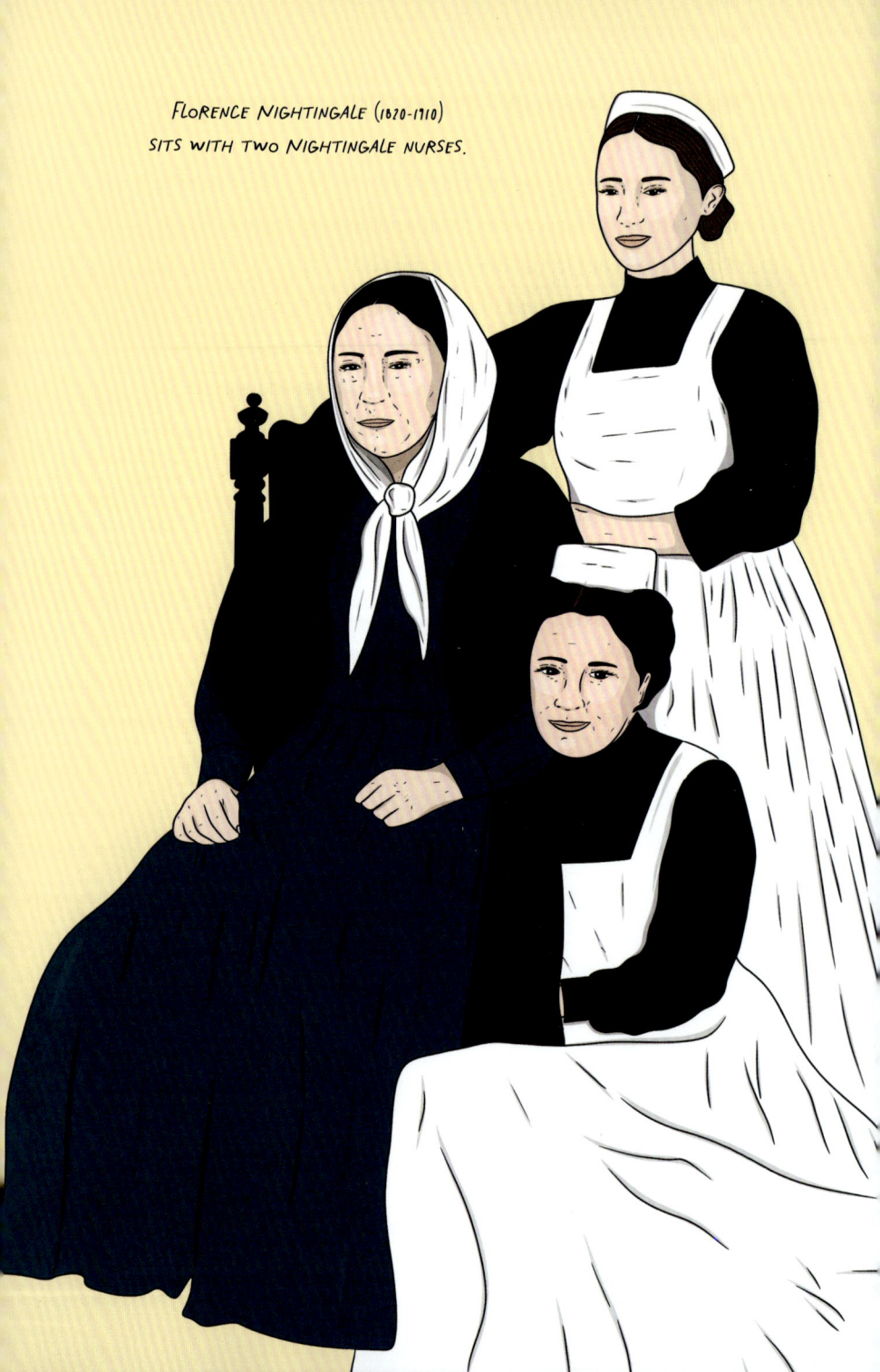

FLORENCE NIGHTINGALE (1820-1910)
SITS WITH TWO NIGHTINGALE NURSES.

CHAPTER NINE

NURSING IN VICTORIAN BRITAIN

When Mary Seacole was in the Crimea, nursing was not yet a respected job. People generally thought that anyone could nurse patients. A nurse's duties mainly involved making up beds, laundry, sewing and cooking.

Florence Nightingale (1820–1910), a wealthy middle-class white woman who was based in the main British hospital at Scutari in Turkey during the Crimean War, played a significant role in making nursing a recognized profession. On her return to England after the Crimean War ended in 1856, Florence Nightingale oversaw many reforms. However, her greatest contribution was helping to change nursing into a 'respectable' profession for middle-class women in Britain.

During this time, it was still rare for people in Britain to go to a hospital for treatment, but this was about to change. Britain had become an **industrial** country. Families had left the countryside to look for work in factories and mines. People flooded into towns and cities, usually living in overcrowded slums, which allowed diseases to spread easily. Medical advances, such as **anaesthetics** and **antiseptic** surgery, also encouraged British people of all classes and backgrounds to come to hospitals when they needed treatment.

As more and more people came to hospitals for treatment, more trained nurses were needed to work in them. In 1860, the Nightingale Training School opened at St Thomas's Hospital in London. Nurses were trained in duties like applying dressings to wounds, bandaging, and applying **leeches**, as well as making beds, cooking and keeping the hospital wards clean. When the Nightingale Training School opened, enslavement throughout the British Empire had already legally ended for more than 20 years. However, the British Empire still existed.

By the start of the First World War in 1914, there were trained nurses in every large hospital in the country. Hospitals used different titles but there were usually four levels of rank for nurses: the most senior nurse was called the matron, below her were the sisters or head nurses, then the staff nurses and finally, the student nurses.

The new-style trained white British nurses did not all remain in the country. Over the next 100 years, thousands of white British nurses travelled to British colonies all over the world.

ASARTO WARD

from Sierra Leone

Asarto Ward was brought to Tottenham, north London in the 1890s from Sierra Leone by Mary Ward (1866–1965). Mary Ward was a white British nurse who worked at the Princess Christian Hospital in Sierra Leone, West Africa from 1892 to 1897.

Before she died, Asarto's mother asked Mary to bring Asarto to England. Asarto was welcomed into the family of Mary's brother, Leonard. When she grew up, Asarto trained to be a nurse at the Prince of Wales's General Hospital in Tottenham. Later on, she returned to Sierra Leone to work in hospitals.

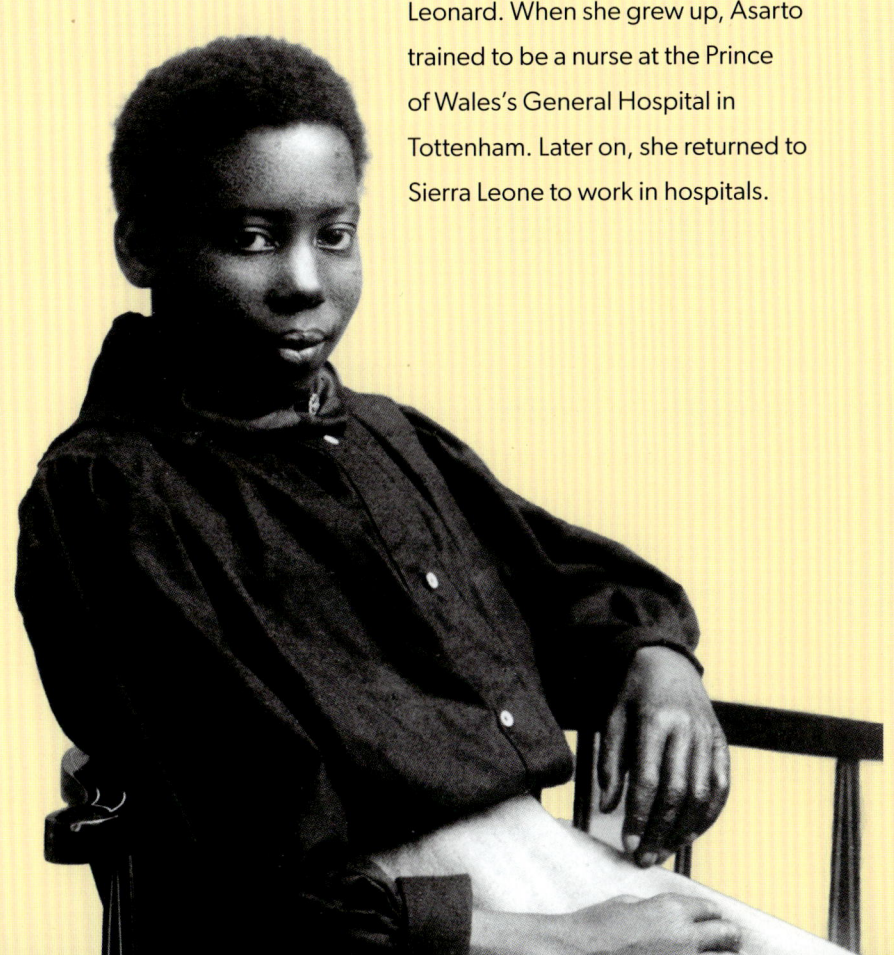

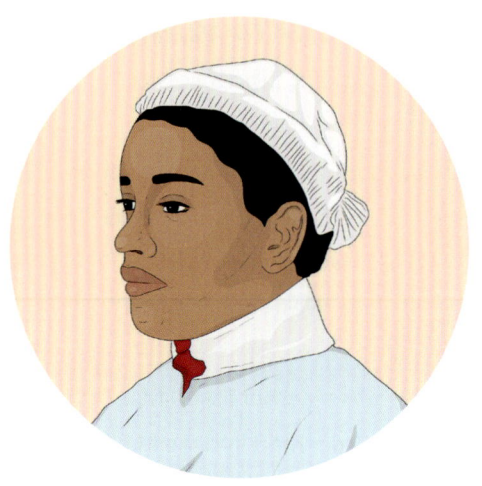

ANNIE CATHERINE BREWSTER
from St Vincent

Annie Brewster was born on the Caribbean island colony of Saint Vincent in 1858. In 1871, Annie and her relatives moved to England.

In 1881, when she was 23 years old, Annie became a student nurse at the London Hospital, located in London's East End – one of just a few places in Britain that had small Black and mixed-race communities.

Annie's record said that she worked well and that '… she was a favourite with all the sisters under whom she worked.' Annie worked at the London Hospital for the rest of her life. When she passed away, the hospital paid for her headstone recognising her '20 years faithful service.'

SARAH WOODBINE
from Argentina

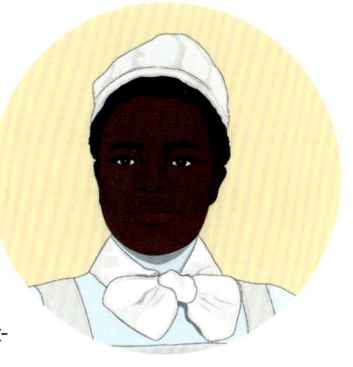

On 8 October 1898, *The Nursing Record & Hospital World* published an article called 'A Plea For Equality' about a Black assistant-nurse in Britain called Sarah Woodbine. The publication recommended Sarah highly and asked British matrons to consider hiring Sarah based on her qualifications. The article outlined Sarah's story of 'determination and courage in spite of many difficulties…'

Sarah came to Britain with her father when she was 14 years old from Argentina because she wanted to train to become a nurse. Sarah wanted to learn the skills to be able to look after her own people: 'They have no one to look after them when ill'. At the time, the white people in Buenos Aires could get trained nurses to look after them.

Sarah was top of the class in her final exams and had found work as an assistant-nurse in a fever hospital. She wanted to be promoted to gain more experience but could not, she said, because of racial **discrimination**. Sarah did not plan to stay in Britain. She wanted to learn how to train student nurses so she would be qualified to train other nurses when she went back to Buenos Aires.

CHAPTER TEN

THE NEW STYLE NURSES GO ABROAD

Almost 30 years after the end of the Crimean War, the leaders of several European countries, the USA and the Ottoman (Turkish) Empire held a meeting in Berlin (in 1884–1885). No African leaders were invited to attend the Berlin Conference. Seven rival European nations, including Britain, divided and claimed most of Africa for themselves.

White British men travelled to Africa as soldiers, settlers and workers to claim 'their' colonies. They set up places to live and work, including hospitals. Usually, separate hospitals were built for white and Black people. The 'European' hospitals were better than the hospitals for Africans. The new-style white British female nurses also travelled out to the African colonies. At first, they went

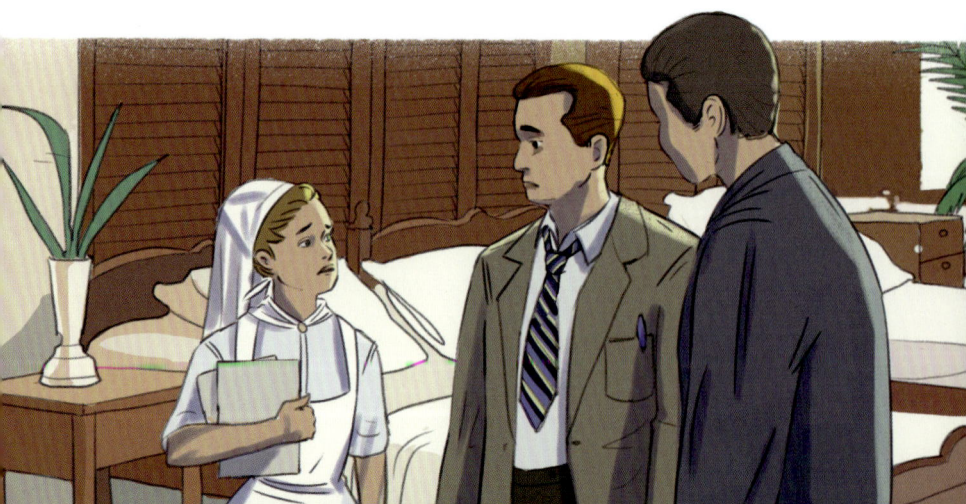

to look after the white British men and their families. Later on, after the First World War ended in 1918, the colonizers began to focus on recruiting Africans to work as nurses too.

By this time, the older colonies in the Americas already had hospitals (see chapter 4). After the enslaved workers were legally freed in the colonies, the sick-houses closed. Public hospitals were opened in most of the colonies. Most were small island colonies and had only one hospital. Unlike in British Africa, these weren't separate hospitals for Black and white people, but some had separate wards that were mainly used by white people. The new-style white British nurses usually went to these colonies to work as matrons and senior nurses.

Nursing abroad gave white middle-class women a chance to travel, earn more money than at home and support the British Empire. The best nursing jobs throughout the empire were kept for white women from Britain. Although there were some Black male doctors by this time, doctors were still usually white men and the senior nurses working with them were expected to be white women.

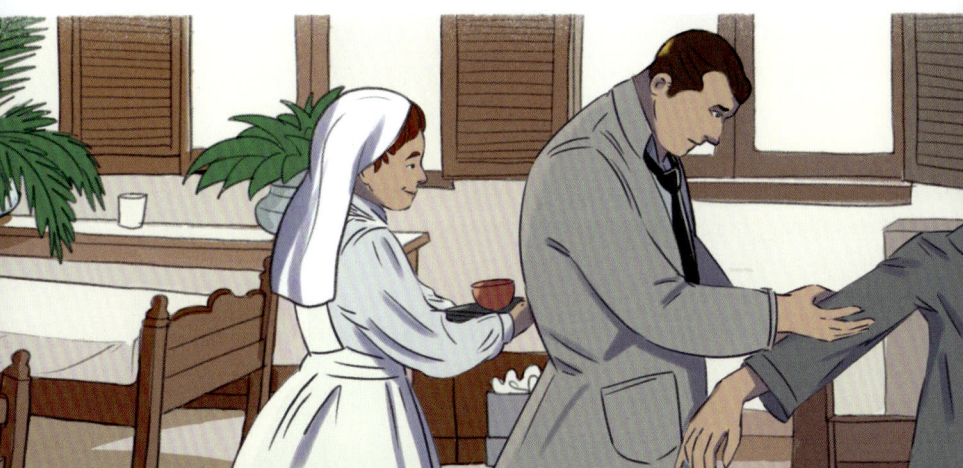

CHAPTER ELEVEN

A COLONIAL WORLD

It wasn't easy for Black women to become new-style trained nurses. Some women in the British colonies travelled to the USA to train as nurses at **segregated** hospitals, such as the Lincoln Hospital in New York. Sometimes they remained in the USA because they couldn't find suitable work in their own countries or elsewhere in Britain and the wider empire.

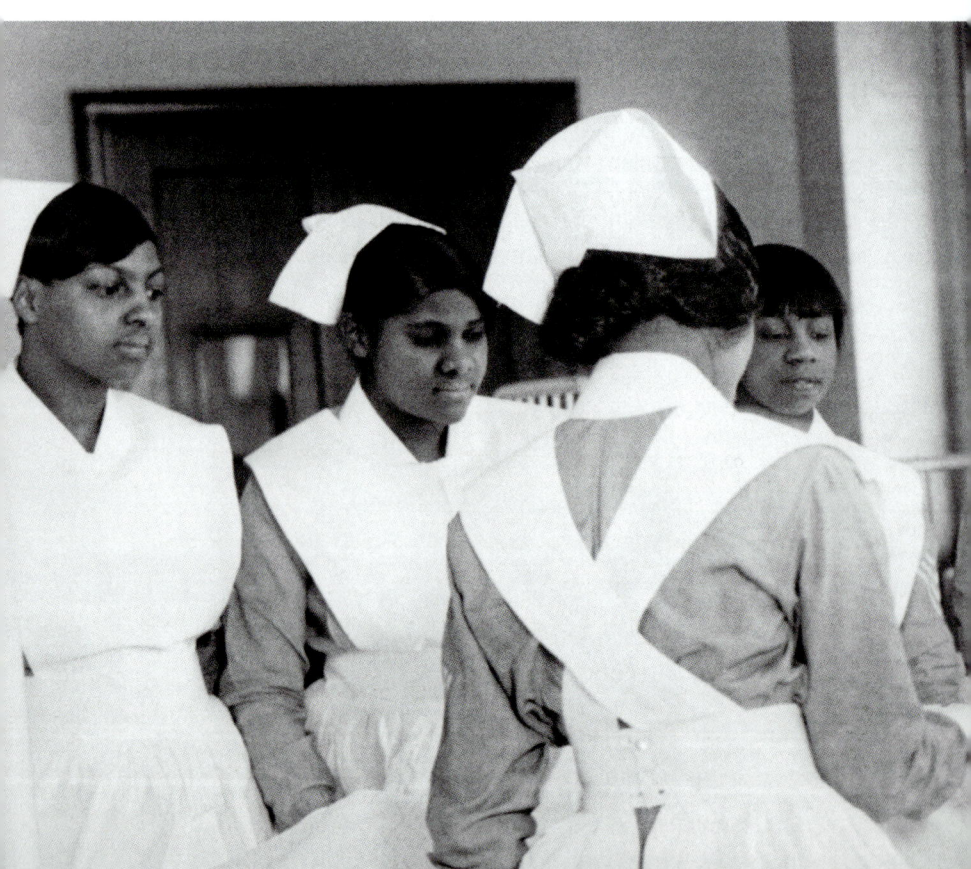

Until the late 1940s, the hospital matron was always a white woman, usually British. The senior nurses were also white, sometimes local white people, white Canadians or white women from other colonies in the region. In some colonies, Black or mixed-race women were allowed to work as hospital nurses. In other colonies, only white women were allowed to be nurses in the hospitals.

THE LINCOLN SCHOOL FOR NURSES IN NEW YORK, USA C1929.
BLACK WOMEN FROM BERMUDA, CANADA, THE CARIBBEAN ISLANDS,
BRITISH GUIANA, THE BAHAMAS AND NIGERIA TRAINED THERE.

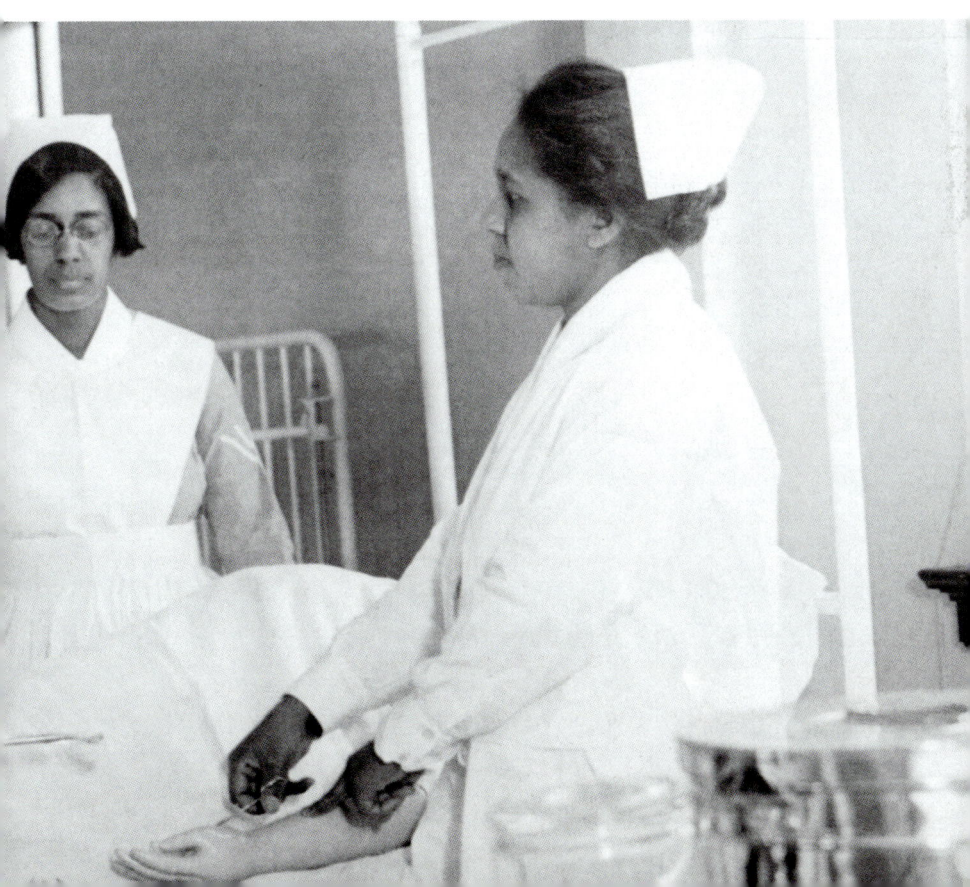

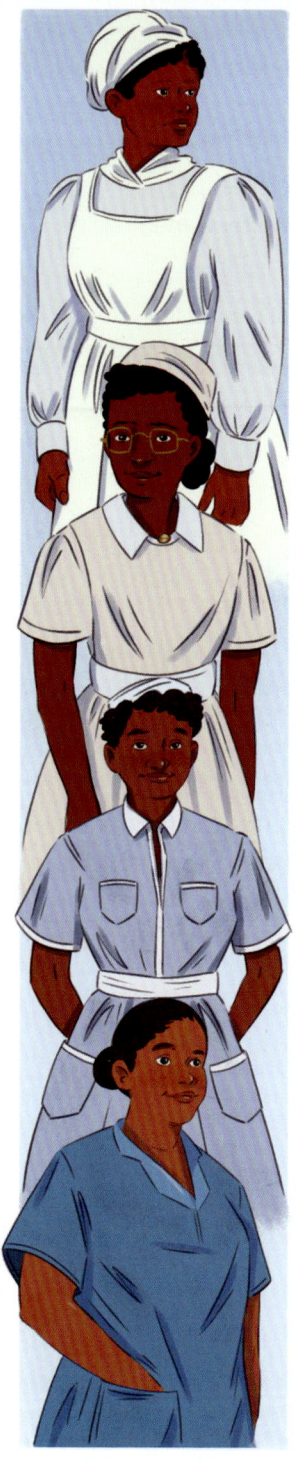

Black nurses had to overcome challenges to find work in hospitals in the British Empire. Some hospitals only wanted to employ British-trained nurses. Others did not accept Black nurses, no matter where they trained. If a trained Black nurse did find work in a hospital, she could never be promoted because the senior nursing jobs in the colonies were kept for white nurses, especially white British nurses. Some trained Black nurses found work outside the colonial hospitals by working privately for wealthy families.

Black Canadian women also found it difficult to become nurses. Until the late 1940s, white Canadians refused to let Black Canadian women attend hospital training schools.

In Africa, the first nurses were often men. As the years went by, more African women became nurses. The men did the nursing work and the female nurses helped them. Nursing training varied from hospital to hospital and colony to colony but could include bandaging, administering medicines and cooking as well as dressing wounds and taking temperatures.

CHAPTER TWELVE

BLACK NURSES IN BRITAIN BEFORE THE 1950s

Before the Second World War (1939–45), Britain was largely white and Christian. Men from various parts of the empire often found work as seamen with Britain's merchant navy. The merchant navy included Africans, Arabs, Caribbeans, Chinese, South Asians and other nationalities. These men often settled in Britain, particularly in seaport towns and cities like London, in the East End, Liverpool, Bristol, Hull, Cardiff and South Shields, but Britain wasn't as diverse as it is today.

It was much rarer for women from the colonies to travel to Britain, especially those who were not white. However like Sarah Woodbine, Black women did continue to come to Britain to try to train and work as nurses. After the Victorian era, some of these student nurses came on scholarships. They didn't come in large numbers and they were expected to leave Britain after they finished their nurse training.

When Britain entered the Second World War, the nurses who were already training and working in hospitals also helped. Lorraine Dyer from Bermuda appeared in a 1943 film along with people from the Caribbean region. The film explained that Lorraine came to Britain from Bermuda in 1937 to train as a nurse and that she would 'open a nursing home when she gets back (to Bermuda)'.

In those days, media was newspapers, radio and films (shown at the cinema). The film was made by the Ministry of Information to be shown to people in the colonies. It gave a good impression of people of different backgrounds working together to help Britain 'fight for victory'. In reality, Black people from the colonies were not encouraged to come to Britain during the war even though many wanted to serve. Eventually, mainly men were allowed to come and most of them served in the Royal Air Force.

Women from Africa also came to Britain to train as nurses during this period. African nurses sometimes came from royal families. Princess Tsahai Selassie and Princess Adenrele Ademola were in Britain during the Second World War and, like Lorraine Dyer, were featured in the media.

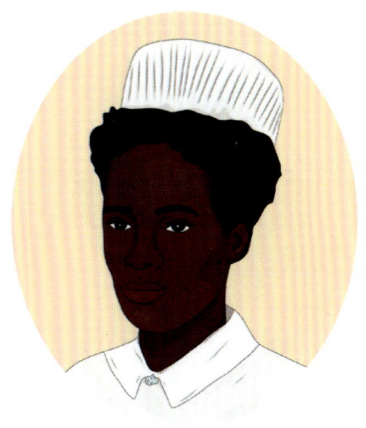

KOFOWOROLA ABENI PRATT

from Nigeria

Kofoworola Abeni Pratt came to Britain in August 1946 to train as a nurse at St Thomas's Hospital in London. Later, she also trained as a midwife. Kofoworola continued her studies and worked as a nurse at Evelina Children's Hospital at Guy's Hospital and at St Thomas's Hospital. She returned to Nigeria in 1954 and became an important nurse leader. In 1964, she became the first Black and Nigerian matron of University College Hospital in Ibadan, Nigeria.

Kofoworola was one of several Black women from Africa and the Caribbean who came to Britain before, during or just after the Second World War to train as nurses. Not only did they help Britain, but those who returned to their home countries often went on to become the first Black senior nurses and matrons in those colonies. This helped to challenge the racism in British colonial society and created change.

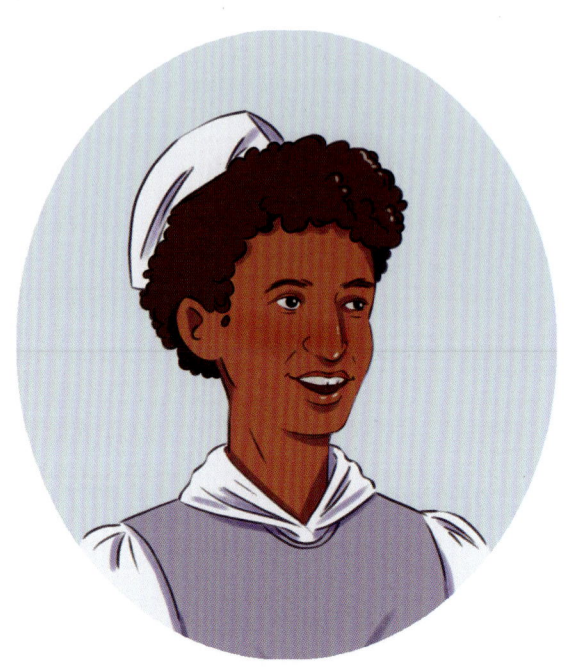

PRINCESS TSAHAI SELASSIE
from Abyssinia (Ethiopia)

In 1941, during the Second World War, the Ethiopian Emperor's eldest daughter who had trained as a nurse at Great Ormond Street, was working at a hospital outside London.

"I TRAINED AS A CHILDREN'S NURSE FIRST. I LOVE CHILDREN. I LOVE YOUR COUNTRY. EVERYONE HAS BEEN SO GOOD TO US."

PRINCESS ADENRELE ADEMOLA

from Nigeria

In October 1941, during the Second World War, Princess
Ademola, daughter of the king of Abeokuta, was training as a
midwife at Queen Charlotte's Maternity Hospital, London. She
intended to return to Nigeria to be involved in the Maternity
Clinics and Child Welfare Centres being established in Abeokuta.

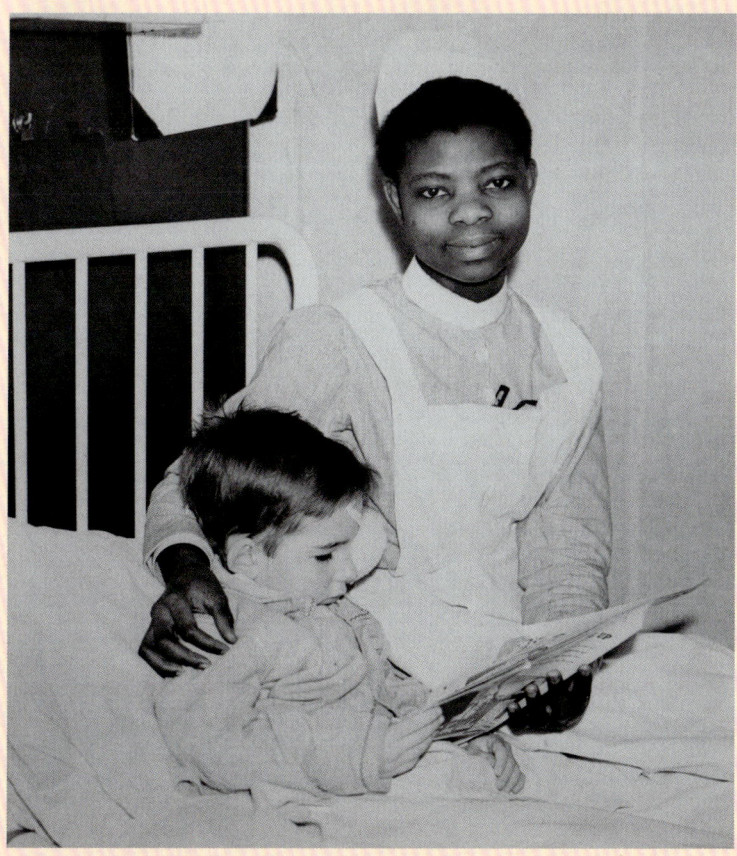

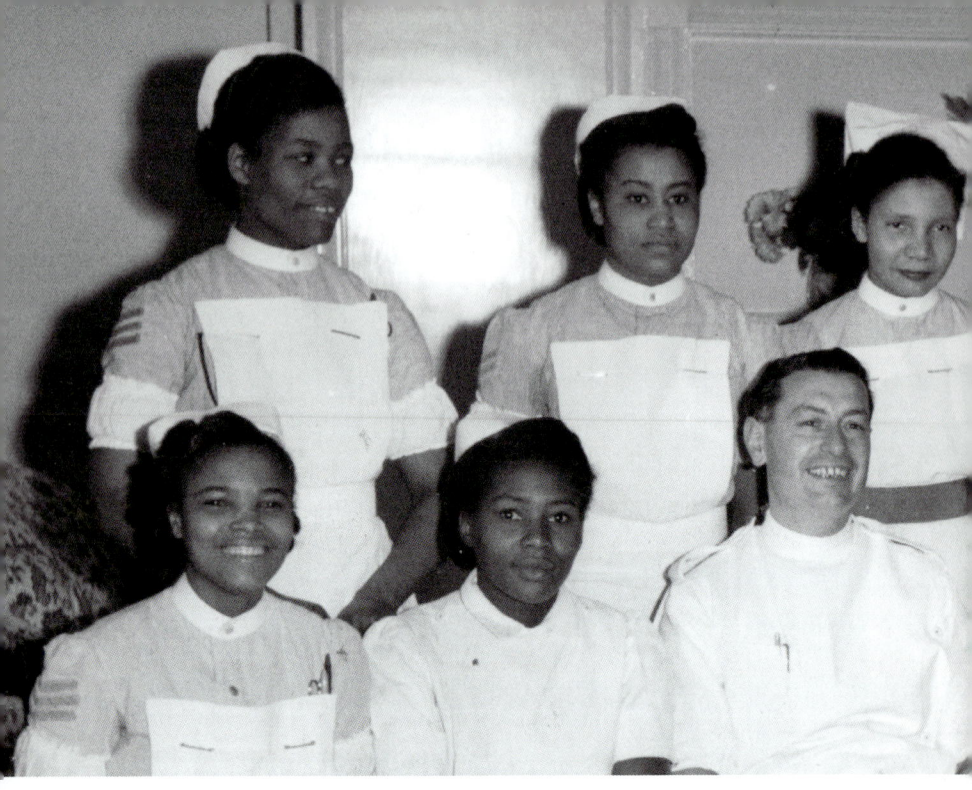

CHAPTER THIRTEEN

BLACK NURSES IN BRITAIN AFTER THE 1950s

In the mid-1950s, large numbers of Black women began to come to Britain to train and work as nurses. Most of them were part of a large-scale movement of people from the colonies in the Caribbean region.

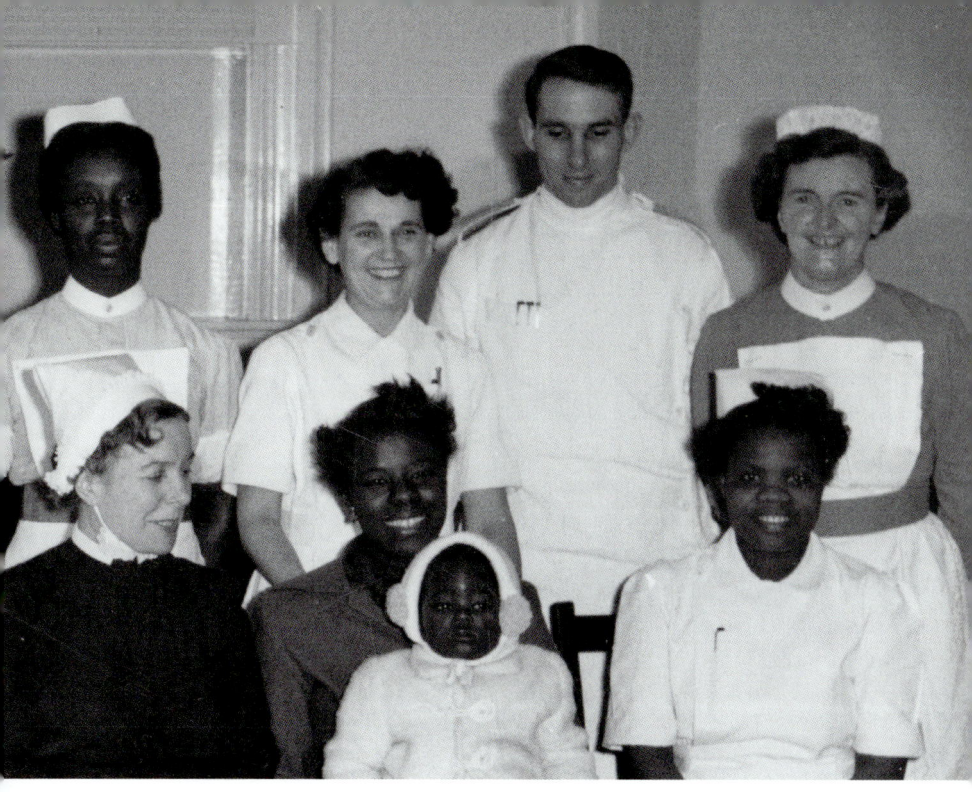

26TH DECEMBER 1953: NURSES AT HACKNEY GENERAL HOSPITAL IN LONDON.

All the colonies in the empire helped Britain achieve its great power and wealth. However, most of the riches benefited the upper classes. Meanwhile, the majority of people in the lower classes had to endure poor living and working conditions.

In the colonies where people of African descent had been enslaved, little had improved in the 100 years since **Emancipation** (when the enslaved were legally freed in 1838). Life was still very difficult.

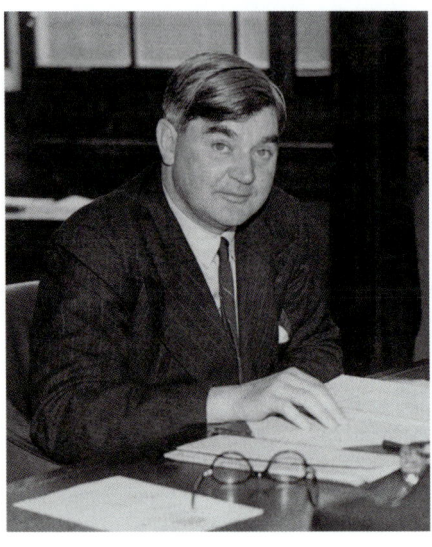

WELSH POLITICIAN ANEURIN
BEVAN (1897-1960), THE NEW
MINISTER OF HEALTH, AT HIS
DESK IN LONDON, AUGUST 1945.

BEVAN WAS THE FOUNDER OF
BRITAIN'S NATIONAL HEALTH
SERVICE (NHS), OFFERING
FREE HEALTHCARE TO ALL
AT THE POINT OF NEED.

People were no longer prepared to accept these wretched conditions. Protests and strikes, which often turned into riots, swept across many Caribbean colonies in the late 1930s including British Honduras (Belize), Trinidad, British Guiana (Guyana), Jamaica, Saint Kitts, Saint Vincent, Saint Lucia, Barbados and Jamaica. Something had to be done!

One of the improvements needed was in healthcare but Britain was engaged in the Second World War from 1939 to 1945 (see chapter 12). After the war ended, more Black women were chosen to come to Britain to train as nurses.

After training in British hospitals, they could return to help improve nursing care in their countries. However, the war had changed things in Britain…

The National Health Service (NHS) was launched in 1948. It was part of a huge plan to improve British society. Before the NHS, most people in the United Kingdom had to pay for medicines, doctors and hospital treatment. The new NHS planned to provide free 'medical, dental and nursing care' to everyone in the UK who needed it, not just those who had money to pay for it. The government planned to raise the money for the service mainly through working people's **taxes**.

However, the new NHS was short of nurses, and other workers, from the start. White British women still became nurses but they were also attracted to secretarial work, teaching and jobs in the civil service. The Ministry of Health, Royal College of Nursing and others began to look for nurses from countries outside the UK. In 1949 they began to look for nurses in the Caribbean too. Nurses came to Britain from many countries including Ireland and Malta.

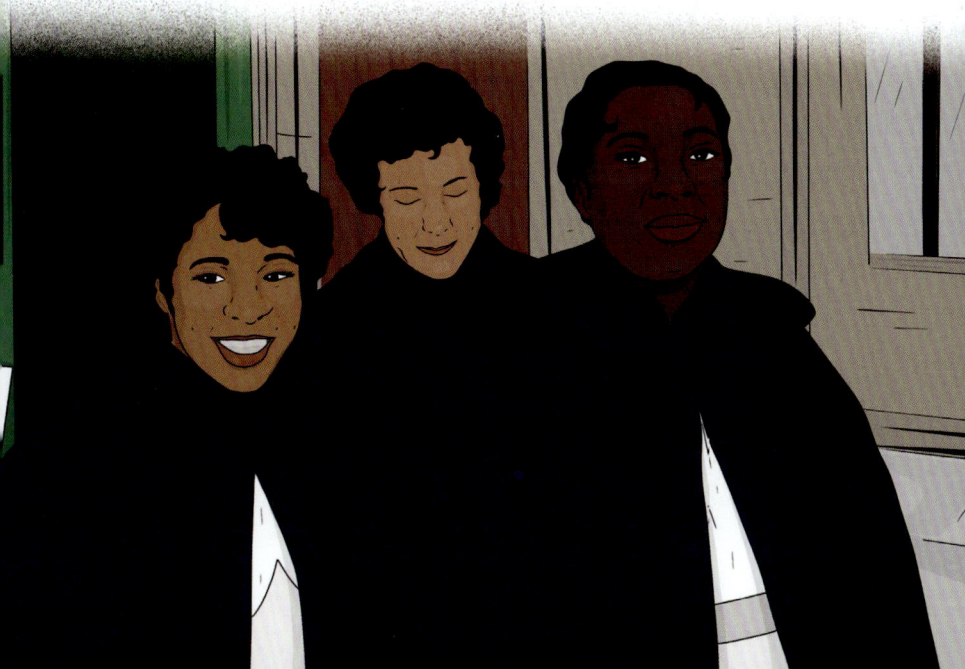

The NHS wasn't the only employer – people also came to work for London Transport, Royal Mail and other organizations but nursing was a popular choice for Black women. Men also came to train and work as nurses. In particular, they worked in hospitals for people with mental illnesses.

Many of the Black nurses came to Britain because they wanted to have a career, learn something new or 'to have an adventure'. Some of them had dreamed of being nurses since childhood. Others wanted to work for the NHS. For most of the young women who were coming to Britain to train as nurses, it was the first time they had left home.

As well as escaping their limited opportunities in the colonies, many Black people were attracted to the idea of 'going to England.' Britain was the capital of the empire and held in high regard. And it was no longer as easy to emigrate to the USA because of recently passed laws there to restrict immigration.

Iris Heard, a white English nurse, began working for the NHS a year after it started;

'When I first got into nursing in 1949 there were just a few girls from West Africa in the hospitals ... They were nearly always from well-to-do families ... Nursing was very low paid in those days.'

After her son had grown up, Iris returned to nursing in the 1960s. She noticed a big change – there were many more Black nurses

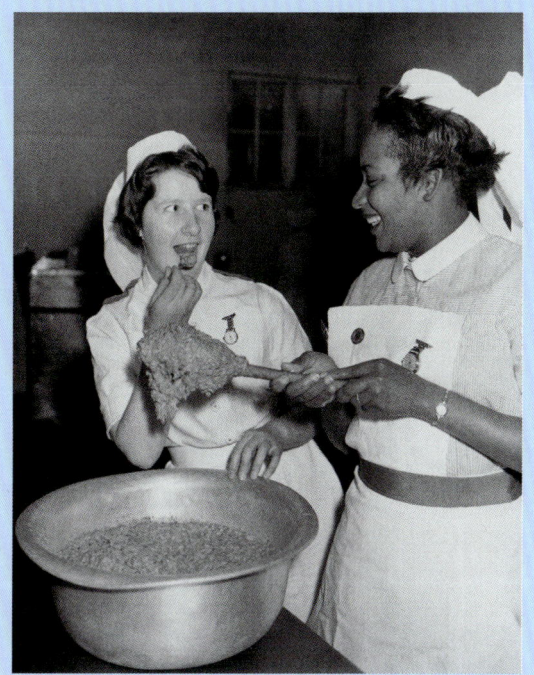

IRISH NURSE THERESA McHUGH TASTES THE CHRISTMAS PUDDING MIXTURE AS BARBADIAN NURSE JULIEN LAUGHS AT WEMBLEY HOSPITAL IN LONDON, UK, 5TH DECEMBER 1960.

in British hospitals and she noticed that they were mainly from the Caribbean.

At first, most of the Black nurses were from the Caribbean colonies but nurses also came from British Africa. Some Black nurses even came from Canada.

Nurses of all backgrounds had to work hard as nursing involved 'long hours, low pay and strict discipline'. Black nurses sometimes also had to cope with discrimination from patients and colleagues. They often were denied equal opportunities for training and promotion.

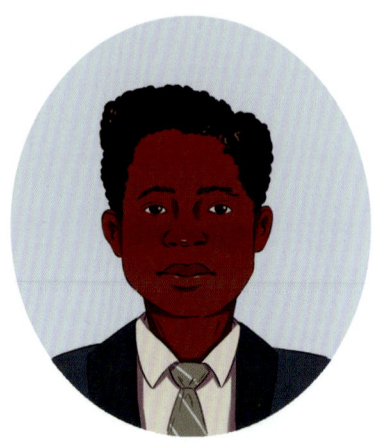

ERIC FERRON

from Jamaica

Most nurses were women, but a few were men. Eric Ferron came to Britain in 1944 from Jamaica and served in the RAF during the war. He remained in Britain and trained as a hospital nurse. At first, Eric didn't want to be a nurse because he thought nursing wasn't a man's job.

Eric felt that things began to change in Britain in 1950. He felt that '… the war was being forgotten' and that 'racism became accepted as a part of the life of the country'. Eric wrote a book about his experiences. He worried greatly about the racial policies in English-speaking countries at the time such as Australia's white-only policy, segregation in some parts of the USA and 'suppression' in South Africa. Eric thought about the links between British colonialism and the issues of the time.

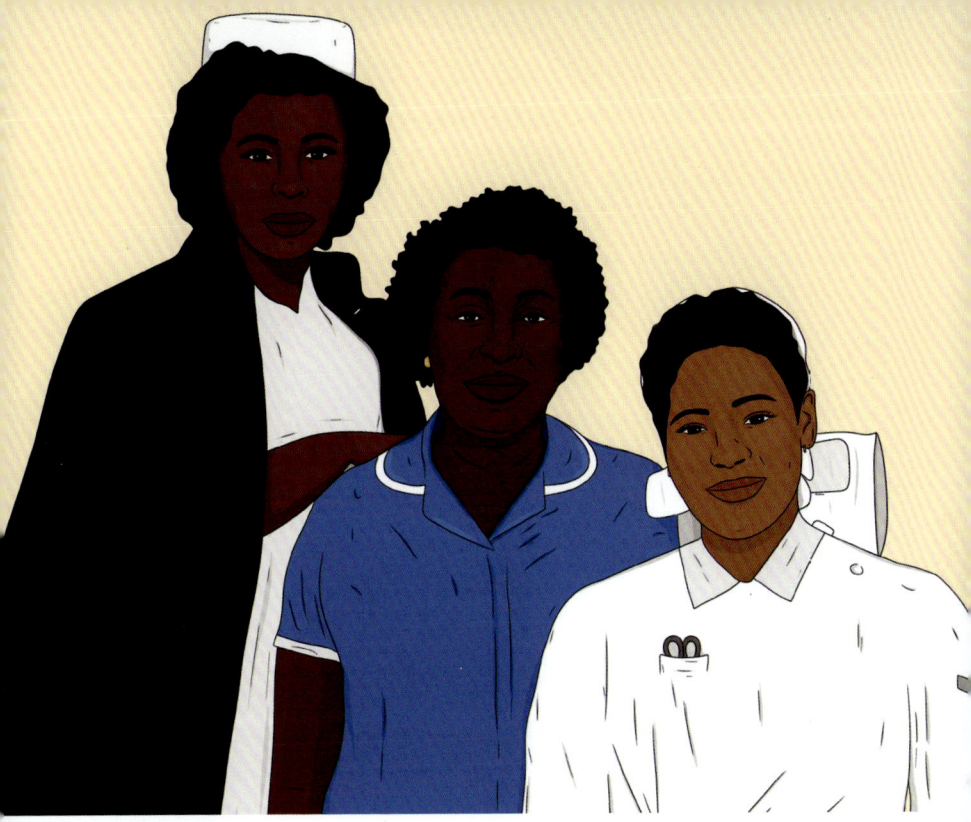

CHAPTER FOURTEEN

A BRIGHTER FUTURE

After working in Britain for some years, some of the Black nurses emigrated again to try to find a better life in countries like the USA and Canada. Others returned to their countries to improve nursing there. As more and more African and Caribbean countries began to break away from the British Empire, many of these women became the first Black matrons and senior nurses in hospitals in their own countries.

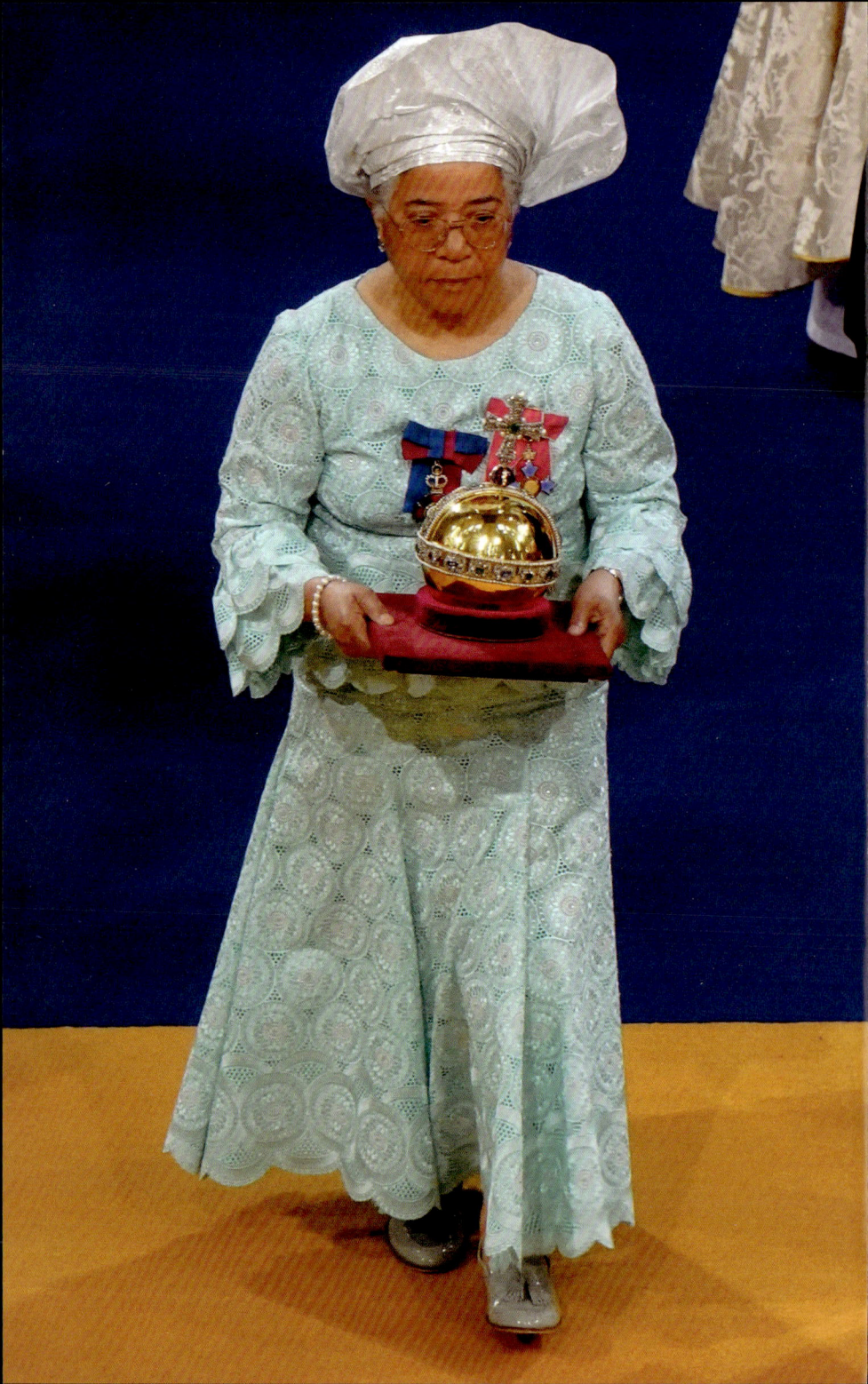

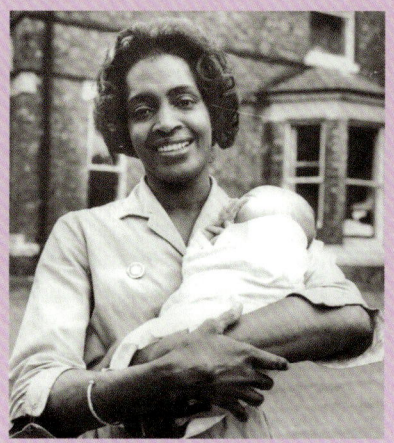

LEFT: *Professor Dame Elizabeth Nneka Anionwu, former nurse, carries the Gold Sovereign's Orb during the Coronation of King Charles III and Queen Camilla on 6th May 2023 in London, England.*

RIGHT: *Daphne Steele was the first black matron of an NHS hospital in Britain.*

Although many left, most of the Black nurses decided to remain in Britain. They continued to contribute mainly by working for the NHS. Daphne Steele from British Guiana (Guyana) made history in Britain when, in 1964, she became matron of the St Winifred's hospital in Ilkley, Yorkshire.

From the 1980s onwards, more Black nurses began to come from Africa. It's hard to believe that Black people were only allowed to train as nurses in large numbers after the Second World War. Today, the NHS workforce is more diverse than ever before. Without Black nurses and healthcare professionals, many hospitals would not have enough staff or expertise to care for patients properly. There are still challenges with discrimination in the job and in the wider society, but they are determined to overcome them so they can continue to help look after us when we need it most.

GLOSSARY

Abolition movement – A long moral and political campaign to outlaw the transportation of enslaved Africans in British ships, and later to free the enslaved people in the colonies.

Americas – Large landmass comprising North America (includes Canada, the USA, Bermuda, the Caribbean and Central America) and South America.

Anaesthetics – Substances that slow or stop the body's ability to feel pain.

Antiseptic – A substance that cleans an area of dirt and germs.

Bankrupt – A person or institution who is unable to pay off their debts.

Cavalry – Soldiers who fight on horseback.

Charms – Objects or spells, which are believed to hold magical qualities.

Cholera – A bacterial disease spread by contaminated food or water. Usually present in areas of poor sanitation and healthcare.

Christopher Columbus (1451–1506) – The first European to establish permanent contact between Europe and the *Americas.*

Colony – A country or geographical area that is under the control of a powerful person, country or government. See also *Empire.*

Discrimination – When a person or group is treated unjustly or with prejudice on the grounds of ethnicity, age, gender or disability.

Empire – A group of peoples and lands under the control of a single person, country or government. See also *Colonies.*

Epidemic – An outbreak of an *infectious disease,* which affects many people in the same place at the same time.

Expedition – A planned journey undertaken by a group for a specific purpose, such as a military operation or research.

Frostbite – A condition where skin is damaged due to exposure to freezing temperatures.

Industrial – Relating to a business or area where lots of goods and products are being manufactured.

Infectious diseases – Diseases, such as measles and colds, which pass easily from person to person.

Leeches – A type of worm that sucks the blood from other animals. Traditionally used by doctors to suck blood from patients in order to 'rebalance' the body's internal workings. Leeches are still used in medicine today.

Lodging-house – An inn, usually in the town, where individuals could rent a room to sleep. Laundry, meals and other services could also be provided.

Malnutrition – A condition where the body does not receive the appropriate nutrients and consequently begins to shut down.

Middle-class – The social group in British society between the working and upper classes. In Britain, this group included doctors and shopkeepers.

Midwife – A medical professional trained to assist in childbirth.

Mummies – Bodies of humans and animals that have been preserved and wrapped in linen bandages.

Natron – A natural type of salt used in ancient times to preserve bodies as part of mummification.

Pharmacist – A medical professional who prepares, dispenses and manages a patient's medications to ensure safe and effective use.

Plantations – A large estate or farm that predominantly cultivates crops such as sugar cane, tobacco or coffee.

Preface – An introduction at the start of a book.

Sanitation – Systems in place to make sure that an area has access to clean water and is free from human waste and other pollutants. A lack of sanitation can lead to disease.

Segregated – When people are separated into more than one group for racial, ethnic or religious reasons.

Sick nurses – People who are tasked with tending to the sick.

Siege – A military operation in which an enemy force tries to convince a town or building to surrender by cutting off its essential supplies.

Smallpox – A viral infection, which causes the sufferer to develop blisters and fever among other symptoms. Eradicated since 1980.

Surgery – A medical procedure in which the body is physically cut open to remove or repair an injured or damaged body part.

Taxes – A mandatory contribution made by an individual or company to the state to help fund the government.

Ventilation – The process of allowing outdoor air to flow through an indoor space, thereby improving air quality.

Yellow fever – An illness transmitted by mosquitoes.

SELECT BIBLIOGRAPHY

Doctors and Slaves, A Medical and Demographic History of Slavery in the British West Indies 1680–1834 by Richard B. Sheridan, Ph.D.

Many rivers to cross: The History of the Caribbean Contribution to the NHS by Ann Kramer

Moving Beyond Borders: A History of Black Canadian and Caribbean Women in the Diaspora by Karen Flynn

In Search of Mary Seacole, The Making of a Cultural Icon by Helen Rappaport

PHOTO CREDITS

QUOTATION CREDITS

Page 8 – Quotation from *The Zambia Nurse*, vol. [1], no. 2, Sept. 1965, p. 1. Women's Studies Archive, the Royal College of Nursing

Page 12 – Quotation from *CARE: 100 Years of Hospital Care in Bermuda* by J. Randolf Williams

Page 16 – Quotation from *Breaking the Glass Ceiling: The Stories of Three Caribbean Nurses* by Jocelyn Hezekiah

Page 20 – Quotation from *No Time for Prejudice* by Mabel Keaton Staupers, R.N.

Page 30 – Quotation from *The Path We Tread* by M. Elizabeth Carnegie

Page 54 – Quotation from *The British Journal of Nursing*, March 1941

Page 60 – Quotation from *Nursing a Nation; An anthology of African and Caribbean contributions to Britain's health services*

ACKNOWLEDGEMENTS

I would very much like to thank the following individuals and institutions for their support, encouragement and help with this book: Sally-Ann Ashton, Virginia Ballance, Stephen Bourne, Audrey Dewjee, Teresa Doherty, Olive Gardner, David Gleave, Debora Heard, Bill Hern, Harriet Pierce, Karen Proverbs, the Royal College of Nursing Library and Archives, Robin Walker and Pedro Welch.

I would also like to thank my friends and family, in particular, Amanda and Dee.

INDEX